Under Quarantine

Under Quarantine

Immigrants and Disease at Israel's Gate

RHONA SEIDELMAN

RUTGERS UNIVERSITY PRESS

NEW BRUNSWICK, CAMDEN, AND NEWARK,
NEW JERSEY, AND LONDON

Library of Congress Catalog in Publication Control Number: 2019008415

ISBN: 978-1-9788-0838-6 (cloth)
ISBN: 978-1-9788-0837-9 (paper)
ISBN: 978-1-9788-0839-3 (ebook)

A British Cataloging-in-Publication record for this book is available from the British Library.

♾ The paper used in this publication meets the requirements of the American National Standard for Information Sciences—Permanence of Paper for Printed Library Materials, ANSI Z39.48-1992.

http://www.rutgersuniversitypress.org

Manufactured in the United States of America

For my family

Contents

Under Quarantine

Barbed Wire

At the heart of this book is a photograph. In 1949, Robert Capa photo-graphed the fence that separated Israel's central immigration camp, Shaar Ha'aliya, from the area around it. There are three people in the picture, with two standing on the outside. They are facing the third individual, who is moving toward them, crawling under the wires. Although the people and their action are at the center of the image, the frame is dominated by the fence itself. We see that this was no small, token barrier. One year after the establishment of the Jewish state and four years after the Holo-caust ended, this image of Israel was dominated by what was a symbol to Jews of European oppression at that time: barbed wire.

This image raises many questions about the motivation for and imple-mentation of so imposing a barrier; about the reactions to it (how it was understood, interpreted, and received); about its failure to act as a deter-rent to the people who crawled under it; and about whether there were consequences to this act of defiance for these new immigrants.

This photograph encapsulates a complex and controversial phenom-enon. Its story and the many questions it raises are at the heart of the his-tory of Shaar Ha'aliya and the quarantine there of Jewish immigrants in the first years of the Jewish state.

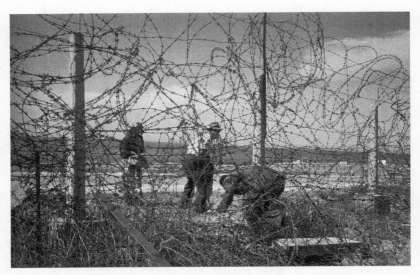

Figure 1. Crawling under the barbed wire fence. © Robert Capa/Magnum Photos.

Not a Quarantine?

Shaar Ha'aliya was the major immigration processing camp in Israel during the period of the mass immigration that followed the establishment of the state in 1948. The central port of entry during an influx of immigration unprecedented in its speed and in its proportion to the residing population, Shaar Ha'aliya was intended to create order by systematizing the social, military, and medical processing that the immigrants were required to undergo. Translated, its name means "gate of immigration."

At first glance, Shaar Ha'aliya comes across as a textbook example of an immigrant quarantine station. Photographs of the camp and historiographical references make it clear that Shaar Ha'aliya was isolated and fenced off and that health concerns played a central role in the camp's conception and function. As a separated space where immigrants underwent medical examinations before entering Israel proper, Shaar Ha'aliya fits well within the definition of quarantine found in the *Oxford English Dictionary* (*OED*):

"A period (originally of forty days) during which persons who might serve to spread a contagious disease are kept isolated from the rest of the community; especially a period of detention imposed on travelers or voyagers before they are allowed to enter a country or town, and mix with the inhabitants; commonly, the period during which a ship, capable of carrying contagion, is kept isolated on its arrival at a port. Hence the fact or practice of isolating such persons or ships, or of being isolated in this way."[1] More important than the OED, the most significant support for the Shaar Ha'aliya / quarantine connection comes from the trove of archival documents that deal with that exact issue. This evidence makes a persuasive case for studying Shaar Ha'aliya's function as a quarantine for Israel's early immigrants.

However, other evidence tells a more complicated story. In the existing literature on mass immigration, Shaar Ha'aliya is referred to in any number of ways: a processing camp, a transit camp, or an immigrant camp.[2] Quarantine does not appear in this variety of terms. Moreover, among some scholars of Israel, there is resistance to the categorization of Shaar Ha'aliya as a quarantine. One individual cautioned that the rhetoric of quarantine must be distinguished from policy and that even if people referred to it as a quarantine, that doesn't necessarily mean it actually was one. Another historian was more forthright in their objection, adamantly asserting that it is historically inaccurate to label Shaar Ha'aliya a quarantine, since their own research shows the State of Israel never quarantined incoming immigrants during the mass immigration.[3]

What makes these reservations particularly intriguing is the many ways they echo the voices coming through in the archival documents. Soon after the establishment of Shaar Ha'aliya in 1949, authorities were immersed in a discussion of its function and perception as a quarantine. The idea that the central port of arrival for Jewish immigrants to the Jewish state could be a quarantine raised passions and resulted in contentious, turbulent debate. Clearly, the contention and disagreement surrounding this issue continue to reverberate into the present day.

Another more tangible point of contention is evident in the archival documents as well: To what extent was the isolation at Shaar Ha'aliya enforced? As we see in Capa's photograph, the barbed wire fence and the police guards at the camp did not actually prevent people from coming in and out. This gap between prescription and practice was known and discussed widely. The Shaar Ha'aliya administration knew that these breaches were a regular occurrence, but they did not see them as an indication that the quarantine was failing and that the barbed wire fence and police could be removed. Instead, they continued paradoxically to insist that the quarantine was necessary to protect the rest of the country from diseases borne by the immigrants.

Axes of Conflict

What can be learned from the many conflicts surrounding the Shaar Ha'aliya quarantine? The lack of consensus, the paradoxes, the level of passion from different quarters—sustained over so many years—all point to the fact that this discussion represents more than just one institution and its health policy: they are valuable indicators of the stakes involved in a medical history of Shaar Ha'aliya.

The story of the Shaar Ha'aliya quarantine is the story of the Israeli immigration experiment, a modern experiment of nation building, belonging, and power that is deeply tied to issues of health and disease. What is at stake is the image and the legacy of Shaar Ha'aliya, the historic gateway for Jewish migration. The conflicts over Shaar Ha'aliya's quarantine are fundamentally about whether Israel's largest, most important "gate of immigration" is understood as a place where Jews were welcomed to Israel or a place where they were made to feel cast out.

We cannot fully understand Israel until we understand Shaar Ha'aliya. Here was the country's crucible. A gateway for nearly half a million immigrants, this is where they began to be changed into the Israeli people and where the Israeli people began to be profoundly changed by them.

The creation of the State of Israel was one of the most transformative events in modern Jewish history. It was established as a homeland and refuge for Jews from across the globe, people who—despite being from vastly different cultures and points of origin—were expected to form an integrated, cohesive nation. As a twentieth-century country striving for normalcy and success within Western standards of its day, Israeli administrators would use tools of modern state building (such as regulation, processing, biomedicine, and quarantine) to try to create a functioning, thriving state. But at the same time, this country was anything but normal. This was a profoundly idealized destination, the Promised Land that people had been praying to and about, yearning for, and imagining and mythologizing for millennia—a homeland that, in the Hebrew lexicon, Jews weren't "immigrating to" but "ascending to"—and that people around the world were scrutinizing and holding up to high expectations. Israel's migrants arrived with a sense of ownership. After a long history of being forced out or refused entry into countries throughout the world—with historically tragic outcomes—here was a country from which Jews would not be turned away. For the majority of the people immigrating to Israel in this time, Shaar Ha'aliya was the gate of entry. It was the first spot in Israel where the historic promise of return was met with the banal realities of bureaucracy and processing, such as impersonal medical examinations and temporary detainment behind barbed wire. The subject of the Shaar Ha'aliya quarantine brings together these emotionally charged and often conflicting foundations of the Israeli experiment in the first years of statehood. It raises questions about how this new and unusual nation of immigrants was actually going to work, what "belonging" was going to look like, and which people and ideas would hold power. This is the phenomenon that the Capa photo encapsulates and that this book examines.

Each chapter explores a different sphere of conflict connected to the Shaar Ha'aliya quarantine: confines, structure, meaning, and memory. "Confines" describes life in Shaar Ha'aliya inside the barbed wire fence. It begins with the larger setting of Israel post 1948, as a way to understand the environment of anxiety into which the immigrants arrived. We will see who came through Shaar Ha'aliya and where they were from. We get a sense of what they experienced in the camp: where they slept, what they ate, who they encountered, how they spent their time. We also learn about the people who worked in Shaar Ha'aliya, many of whom were also immigrants. And finally, we will learn about the function of health services in the camp, the medical examinations the immigrants went through, and the story of the Institute for the Treatment of Ringworm and Trachoma in Immigrant Children, a separate and controversial medical facility that opened in Shaar Ha'aliya in 1952. As will be discussed, Western medicine's standard treatment for ringworm in the 1950s was a painful procedure involving waxing and tweezing the patient's head and then treating the bald surface with radiation. Historically, children with ringworm were often isolated from others for extended periods, which is part of what happened at the Ringworm and Trachoma Institute in Shaar Ha'aliya. The traumatic and painful medical procedure in the 1950s, the extended separation from families at the treatment institute, the fact that the majority of children who were treated for this ailment at Shaar Ha'aliya were from Arab and Muslim countries, and then the prevalence of head and neck tumors that appeared in later years among people who had been treated there as children have come together to leave an open wound in Israeli society. The Shaar Ha'aliya Institute for the Treatment of Ringworm and Trachoma in Immigrant Children is at the center of this wound. Its history, and the broader context provided in this chapter, clarify the camp's particular medical and social role while shedding light on the many challenges that were a part of life in Israel and in Shaar Ha'aliya itself.

"Structure" focuses on the physical struggle for control of the quarantine: the construction of the fence, the ways the immigrants physically defied it—by breaking in and out—and the administration's ambivalent responses. This chapter puts quarantine in historical context, as a way to understand the development of this phenomenon, particularly in Western medicine, in Palestine and Israel. This contextualization helps explain why a central camp for the quarantine of immigrants would have a place in the modern State of Israel, and it helps us understand how it could be so brazenly disregarded by new immigrants. We will see that the fence at Shaar Ha'aliya was not only a structure of confinement but also a site of negotiation and a vehicle for immigrant rebellion and empowerment. This section ties in with the work of scholars such as Orit Rozin, Bryan K. Roby, and Orit Bashkin who increasingly emphasize the importance of immigrant rebellion in the experience of the mass immigration.

"Meaning" moves from the physical into the realm of ideas and relates to the conflicts surrounding how the Shaar Ha'aliya quarantine looked and seemed. I focus on the different interpretations that people had of the fence and the images of Israel that it conveyed. For some, it was a comfort, a measure that suggested security, keeping the perceived dangers of disease and immigration at bay. For others, it was an infuriating and shameful symbol of isolation that threatened the social fabric of the new society. This chapter speaks to the tremendous power of what historian Alan M. Kraut has called the "double helix" of health and immigration—two themes that remain inextricably linked and powerfully shape the way absorbing societies see new immigrants.[4] I argue that the only way to understand the contradictions in the defense of Shaar Ha'aliya's quarantine, which was being touted as medically necessary by the same people who knew that men, women, and children were coming and going through holes in the fence, is through the contexts of Israeli and medical history. This idea of quarantine is directly influenced by the power of fear, fences, and twentieth-century medicine. For the people who defended it, quarantine meant an authoritative and familiar solution, even when it was, in fact, irrational. To many people in what was known as the "Yishuv"[5]—the greater Israeli, Jewish society—it suggested a sense of control in this period of dramatic change, uncertainty, and fear.

"Memory" steps away from the past to discuss the contemporary marginalization of Shaar Ha'aliya in Israeli historiography and in Israel's official public remembrances, shedding light on why the association between Shaar Ha'aliya and quarantine could, to many, still be considered problematic. The conflict here is between the numerous and rich personal remembrances of Shaar Ha'aliya, its quarantine, and the state's omission of this story. I claim this is an intentional omission because the many remembrances of Shaar Ha'aliya that do exist destabilize a few central—and comfortable—hegemonic Zionist narratives that actively construct nationhood: Jewish victimhood; the heroic struggle against an "external" oppressor; the myth of immigration that is Zionist, vulnerable, and heroic; and the myth that medicine is purely benevolent and healing. I begin the discussion of memory and remembrance through a comparison with the memorialization at Atlit. The site of this former detention camp, where illegal Jewish immigrants to Mandate Palestine were held behind barbed wire by British authorities, is located only a few miles from the historic site of Shaar Ha'aliya. While there is not even a sign at Shaar Ha'aliya explaining what this place once was, at Atlit, there is an elaborate heritage museum that prominently features barbed wire as a symbol of Britain's cruel containment of the Jewish refugees. Yet the themes that are so importantly a part of Israel's official memorialization of Atlit are similar to the remembrances of Shaar Ha'aliya that we find in memoirs, oral testimony, and art. As such, this chapter sheds light on how the memory of Shaar Ha'aliya and its medically defended barbed wire challenge a mythic narrative of Israel. An important part of this chapter is the traumatic remembrance of ringworm treatment at Shaar Ha'aliya and the mark it has left on contemporary Israeli society.

I end my discussion in 1952 because this is the year that the number of immigrants to Israel and Shaar Ha'aliya significantly declined, as a result of the selective immigration policy that was adopted by the Israeli government in November 1951. As historian Avi Picard has shown, selective immigration was a controversial idea that was accepted largely because of health concerns associated with the mass immigration. As a result, 1951 marks the end of the first and largest wave of Israel and Shaar Ha'aliya's post-1948 immigration.[6] These factors join together to give a discussion on immigration, health, and quarantine in the years 1949 to 1952 a particular urgency and salience.

HISTORIOGRAPHY AND THE MIZRAHI/ASHKENAZI DIVIDE

Historians began to look to Israel's mass immigration as a valuable field of exploration in the late 1990s. In her groundbreaking work *Immigrants in Turmoil*, historian Dvora Hacohen was the first to use archival research to show the complex absorption system into which the new immigrants arrived and the numerous obstacles they faced upon their arrival.[7] Recent scholars have built upon this foundation, making important advances in the writing of social and medical histories of 1950s Israel and working to incorporate the perspectives of the immigrants themselves. These invaluable studies have turned a critical eye on state hegemony and systems of power and, accordingly, have put to rest any simplistic or romantic notions of Israel's "Ingathering of the Exiles." Much of this newest historiography focuses on the experiences of particular ethnic and immigrant groups.[8] Others map the Israeli policies—as well as medical, technological, cultural, and social norms—that shaped the period and impacted both the immigrant's arrival and the immigrant-Israeli encounter.[9]

Under Quarantine follows in the tradition of this critical turn in Israeli medical and social history. This book is deeply influenced by research that has animated and complicated our understanding of the history of Israel's formative years. Where *Under Quarantine* departs from other scholarship on this period is in its focus on this one pivotal place and its role in Israel's origin story. In doing so, it aims to bring Shaar Ha'aliya—and the immigrant experience there—out of the margins of historiography and public remembrance. This book looks at Shaar Ha'aliya as a conduit, unlike any other in Israel, where the particular histories, policies, and norms come together. And it looks at Shaar Ha'aliya's fence as a microcosm that brings to the surface some of the most crucial issues concerning the history of Israel and its migrants. Furthermore, by choosing to examine Shaar Ha'aliya

through the discipline of medical history, this book allows us to contextu-
alize the phenomenon of this camp and its quarantine within a broader,
global frame. For although Shaar Ha'aliya is most directly about Israel, the
currents that shape its story—migrants, contagion, isolation—are by no
means unique to Israel.

In making its argument, this book moves away from the Ashkenazi/
Mizrahi dichotomy that often sets the frame for discussion of Israel's first
years.[10] In Shaar Ha'aliya, the common themes of racism and ethnocen-
trism toward Mizrahim (Jews of North African or Middle Eastern origin) versus Ashkenazim (Jews of mostly Central and Eastern European
origin) are too cut and dry. Orit Bashkin's complication of the ubiquitous term *Mizrahi* is valuable for understanding this issue. In *Impossible
Exodus: Iraqi Jews in Israel*, Bashkin emphasizes the cultural and linguis-
tic diversity of the various groups who fall under this label, making the
important argument that we need to "break the more general category
of 'Mizrahim,' in order to explore the histories and identities of specific
Middle Eastern countries in Israel."[11] Bashkin then shows that the Mizrahi
identity developed later in the Israeli immigration experience as a result
of the struggle against Ashkenazi hegemony.[12] Eventually, the immigrants
came to see that there were some problems that immigrants from North
African and Middle Eastern countries had in common: poverty, poor
access to quality education, housing problems, low-income jobs.[13] It was
from this difficult Israeli experience that the Mizrahi identity emerged.[14]
With this in mind, we can understand that—in fact—there were no Mizrahim in Shaar Ha'aliya. There were immigrants from countries including Iraq, Iran, Egypt, Tunisia, and Morocco for whom, eventually, *Mizrahi*
would become an additional dimension of who they were. For many, this
identity formation began at Shaar Ha'aliya. But in Shaar Ha'aliya itself,
the Mizrahi identity had not yet been forged.

Another factor complicating the Ashkenazi/Mizrahi dichotomy is the
fact that Holocaust survivors—who went through Shaar Ha'aliya in large
numbers and had an important place in the Yishuv's image of the mass

immigration—were also viewed by the Yishuv as diseased and potentially socially contaminating. A topic that surfaces repeatedly throughout
this book is how the immigrants' various ethnic backgrounds and their
encounters with stereotyping and discrimination shaped their Israeli experience in various ways—both in and outside of Shaar Ha'aliya. However,
my conclusion is that this camp and its quarantine were not expressly
intended to target one ethnic group more than another. In this respect
at least, the people who went through Shaar Ha'aliya were bound by the
commonality of being immigrants.

As the details of this story will show, Shaar Ha'aliya affected individuals differently. At this first moment of arrival, the large categorizations of
Mizrahi and Ashkenazi are not a reliable way to understand whether a
person would have felt welcome or happy or discriminated against and
traumatized. Some North Africans were deeply scarred by their time there,
while others hardly remember it. Some Europeans were unmoved by what
they found there, while for others, the camp conjured memories from the
war and the Holocaust. One man who was there for weeks considered it
"fine," while others who were there for several hours considered it horri-
ble. How one experienced Shaar Ha'aliya was largely an individual matter,
the outcome of the interaction between factors of language, background,
time, lodgings, food, weather, interpersonal relations, age, expectations,
and past experience that resulted in one's own personal encounter and
memories.

MIGRATION, ISRAEL

This book is about the extraordinary phenomenon of mass migration. It
celebrates the migrants whose incredible lives form the heart of the story.
Today, our early twenty-first-century world is being transformed by the
largest mass migrations in recent history, with expansive immigrant and
refugee camps appearing across the globe, as well as walls and medical-
ized, nativist rhetoric and policy. In such a world, Shaar Ha'aliya's story

is more important than ever. We will see the upheaval that mass migrations bring to everyone involved and the various ways different people cope with this upheaval. We will see the exceptional difficulties a person encounters when reaching a new country, the practical challenges a society faces when trying to accommodate new immigrants, and how deeply vulnerable people can feel when immigrants arrive at their borders. This is a story that helps us understand how those vulnerabilities can both connect to and exaggerate the fear of illness and disease. It helps us understand the important role that medicine plays in controlling migrants. And finally, it helps us see how these fears—of foreigners, of contagion—can lead to quarantine being used to rationalize an exclusion even when it is not medically justifiable.

For Israel, the significance of Shaar Ha'aliya cannot be overemphasized. It has no parallel in Israeli history. Although in various stages of the mass immigration there were other areas of controlled immigration centers,[15] Shaar Ha'aliya was the only central processing camp. In its thirteen years of operation, nearly 400,000 immigrants passed through its gates, with the overwhelming majority (325,296) concentrated in 1949–1952.[16] By 1952, approximately one quarter of the entire Israeli population had immigrated by way of this camp. Some of these individuals went on to become famous cultural and political figures, including the celebrated author Eli Amir, the singer Chava Alberstein, as well as the disgraced former president Moshe Katzav. As we will see, Shaar Ha'aliya shaped Israeli culture, the Israeli landscape, and Israeli society. The Jewish Agency conceived of it as an isolated space where the masses could be met, contained, and controlled with order. But in so many ways, the immigrants who went through Shaar Ha'aliya defied this balance of power. The people who emerged from this flawed process were emboldened, often disappointed, and vocally and physically defiant and carried with them a strong sense of entitlement to the goings-on in their state. In the controlled chaos of the Shaar Ha'aliya tents, huts, lines, and fence, we can see the people, and the newly complicated encounters between people, that were bringing Israel to life.

A "Broader Applicability" of Quarantine

Shaar Ha'aliya's history pushes the boundaries of what is and what is not considered a quarantine. In 1948, Israel had three official, functioning quarantine stations for international travelers, at the Haifa, Tel Aviv / Jaffa, and Eilat ports. Shaar Ha'aliya was not one of them.[17] Historian Dan Bar-El has shown that modern quarantine systems for travelers to Palestine were introduced as part of international initiatives to control the spread of cholera in the nineteenth century. The first quarantine station in Jaffa was opened in 1835, following the second cholera outbreak in the region. European consulates wanted to closely supervise this main entry to the Holy Land.[18] Medical historian Nissim Levy explains that under the British rule of Palestine (1917–1948), quarantine for travelers faded from use and significance.[19]

According to Theodor Grushka's foundational manuscript on Israeli public health, in 1948, the diseases listed as "quarantinable" were smallpox and louse-borne typhus.[20] Although there had been a few minor outbreaks of smallpox in 1949–1950, internationally accepted vaccination procedures prevented any recurrence.[21] Indeed the "great quarantine diseases of smallpox, plague and cholera, when they did occur, were limited to small foci and quickly stamped out."[22] From 1948 to 1965, Israeli public health services did not receive any reports of quarantinable diseases, nor were any registered in vessels coming in to Israel.[23] Nissim Levy goes on to assert that once the State of Israel was established, the entire institution of quarantine "was left off and completely forgotten."[24]

With this in mind, anyone who argues that Shaar Ha'aliya was not a quarantine is not entirely wrong. It was outside the equation of international quarantine stations that can be framed so precisely. But this definition falls flat: it is limited and superficial. Foucault famously exposed the blurred boundaries between quarantine and other forms of state-imposed isolation and punishment.[25] Carolyn Strange and Alison Bashford have continued Foucault's comparative approach, asking us to see what is uniquely modern about isolating practices. They have identified three vital characteristics: (1) flexible rationales for the isolation that "often move seamlessly between punishment, protection and prevention," (2) architectural dimensions that have been carefully planned out, and (3) the "subjectification of the isolated."[26]

If we look at quarantine in this way—as a modern method of enforced isolation, with shifting rationales for confinement, a careful architectural structure that is a place where the people inside are not only subjectified but also objectified—we find, almost precisely, a definition of Shaar Ha'aliya. Here, in the modern State of Israel, was a camp that was, to a large extent, being defined by an architectural structure: its fence. But the rationale for what it was and why it needed to be separate (because it was a quarantine, an immigration camp, or a processing camp?) is still, to this day, rather slippery. And the people inside, as we will see, were powerful subjects. This insight helps us see Shaar Ha'aliya's quarantine as something that fits within a global process of modernization.

Other scholars of quarantine give us an opportunity to strip the concept down and understand it more fully as a basic, emotional, human act of separation and not only as an explicit public health policy. It is a disruption of contact.[27] It is a boundary. It is a way to put distance between people who are contaminating and people who are uncontaminated.[28] But as medical historian David Musto cautions, in the history of quarantine, "social diseases"—including the "disease" of immigration, drugs, and feared minorities—have always been targeted as much as biological disease. Accordingly, he calls for a wide perspective: "The concept of quarantine is far broader than its modern applicability to a well-understood communicable disease. Quarantine is a marking off, the creation of a boundary to ward off a feared biological containment lest it penetrate a healthy population."[29] This is where we find Shaar Ha'aliya, within this "broader applicability" of quarantine. Shaar Ha'aliya was not necessarily one of Israel's official international quarantine stations but—as we will see—neither was it just a metaphor for quarantine. In a time of deep existential anxiety for citizens of a vulnerable new country, during an extraordinary wave of mass migration, it was a boundary meant to "ward off" the "disease" of immigration, separating the (physically and socially) contaminating from the uncontaminated. But because the people it was meant to ward off were the same people that Israel was said to be welcoming—the same people Israel was meant to be *for*—it was perhaps inevitable that this "warding off" would not go unchallenged. It was fundamentally provocative from the start.

CHAPTER 1

Confines

FACING THE MASS IMMIGRATION, 1948–1952

To mark the opening of Shaar Ha'aliya in March 1949, Yehuda and Leah Weisberger put on nice clothes, stood formally beside one another, and had their picture taken next to a sign stuck in the sand. It read as follows: The Jewish Agency of Israel / Absorption Department / Shaar Ha'aliya Processing Camp / Haifa. This was a big day for the Weisbergers. After years of having various appointments in the Jewish Agency, gaining experience and moving his way up the ladder, Yehuda was poised to begin the job of a lifetime, director of Israel's Ellis Island. Since his wife, Leah, was a trained nurse, she would also have an important role to play in the camp, overseeing health care programs for children and new mothers. It was clear to Yehuda that he and Leah were taking part in something historic. He had come to Palestine, alone, when he was nineteen years old, to escape virulent anti-Semitism in his native Poland. Now here he was thirteen years later. His father and sisters had been murdered only a few years earlier, along with almost all the Jews of Europe; and he was standing next to his wife in the Jewish state about to take part in what he described as "the incredible enterprise of the Ingathering of Israel's Exiles."[1] Shaar Ha'aliya was going to be the main artery through which Israel's hundreds of thousands of new immigrants would enter; and Yehuda, a thirty-two-year-old man in glasses, a suit, and a tie, was going to be directly responsible for them all.

At this time, everything around Yehuda and Leah was quickly changing. The Jewish state that they had dreamed about and worked toward had finally become a reality. Yet not even a year had passed since its independence, and it was far from clear whether this country would be able to overcome its many, very serious problems. In those months between Israel's declaration of statehood in May and the Weisbergers' Shaar Ha'aliya photograph in March, the 1948 war had racked their surroundings with horrifying violence, instability, and explosive demographic transformations. Six thousand Jews—a full 1 percent of the Jewish population of Israel—had been killed in the war. Between 6,000 and 12,000 Palestinian Arabs were killed in that same conflict, and another 750,000 had become stateless refugees living outside of Israel's borders. In March 1948, a year before the Weisbergers had their photograph taken, Palestinian Arabs had made up the majority of the population of British Mandate Palestine, numbering more than 1,000,000 people. When Yehuda and Leah posed for the opening of Shaar Ha'aliya, there were only 150,000 Palestinian Arabs—now Arab citizens of Israel—within the new borders of the Jewish state. Israel recognized the remaining Palestinians as citizens of the country. But the wounds of the violent 1948 war were fresh and remained deeply unresolved. There was deep distrust and distance between the Arabs and Jews of Israel. The Israeli state put the Arab minority under military rule and turned its attention to its main priority: taking in Jewish refugees and immigrants from across the globe.[2]

Today we know that the outcome of the war was actually well-suited to the balance of military and political power: Israel was the stronger side and that is why it won the war. But this was far from what the public knew in 1948 and 1949, so Yehuda and Leah would almost certainly have felt what the majority of Israelis and Jews throughout the world were feeling: this was a David and Goliath story, with one Jewish state attacked by five Arab states; it was almost miraculous that Israel had survived the war; and it was amazing that so soon after the Holocaust Jews would finally have a country that they could turn to for refuge, a country that, unlike most others, would not turn them away.[3]

What followed is what is known as the mass immigration. Between May 1948 and January 1952 nearly seven hundred thousand Jews moved to Israel, more than doubling the Jewish population in only a few short years. Modern Jewish immigration to Palestine had begun at the end of the nineteenth century. From 1882 to 1948, over the course of sixty-six years—through Ottoman and then British rule of the land—hundreds of thousands of Jews moved to Palestine, primarily from Eastern and Central Europe, joining the Jewish minority and Arab majority that had been living there for generations.[4] The first immigrants to the State of Israel, the people of the mass immigration, were from more than thirty vastly different countries in Eastern and Western Europe, the Middle East, and North Africa.[5] Their stories are of separation from homes, distance from the familiar, uprooting, relocation, and the struggles of growing new attachments and roots. For some, moving to Israel was an inspired act, infused with messianic significance: the return to the Holy Land. For some, it was an act of nationalism, the identification with, and desire to be a part of, political Zionism. For others, it was the last resort after being left with no nationality and no other potential asylum. All were coping with adjusting their hopes and expectations to the harsh realities of foreignness and reconstruction.[6]

Bringing Jewish immigrants to Israel was of paramount priority to the new state. Before the 1930s, many Zionist leaders—most notably David Ben-Gurion—had preferred for Jews to come to Palestine through a process of selective immigration. The candidates for immigration would be prepared and educated before arriving, ensuring that when they did arrive, they would be well suited to contribute to the Zionist mission. But with growing anti-Semitism in Europe, preparing Jews abroad and then bringing them in slowly was no longer a privilege Zionists could afford: the situation was becoming increasingly perilous and there were fewer and fewer countries where the persecuted Jews of Europe could turn for sanctuary. Historian Dvora Hacohen writes that in 1939, after the horrific pogroms of Kristallnacht had shattered "any illusions there may have been about the Nazi regime" and the British authorities had restricted Jewish immigration to Palestine with the White Paper of 1939, "there was a growing sense of helplessness and alarm in the *yishuv*."[7] Things became more desperate when, in April 1943 at the Bermuda Conference between England and the United States, the superpowers "decided that Jewish refugees could not be brought out of occupied Europe because no country would have them."[8] Faced with this grim reality and the limited power Jews held in British-controlled Palestine, Hacohen asks, "How could they fight? What means did [Ben-Gurion] have at his disposal?"[9] The answer was immigration. Ben-Gurion imagined a "rebellion of immigration."[10] This meant two important things: lives would be saved and the Jewish national homeland would increase its Jewish population. From then on, facilitating unrestricted, mass immigration of Jews to Palestine, and then to Israel, thus became a top priority for the Zionist movement and then a central policy of the state, which set the stage for the mass immigration.[11]

People like Yehuda and Leah Weisberger, who were part of the largely Ashkenazi "veteran"[12] absorbing population, were excited about the realization of a Jewish state and the utopian ideal behind the mass immigration, the "Ingathering of the Exiles" that envisioned the Zionist state drawing in and embracing all Jews seeking shelter.[13] But they were also deeply unsettled by the immigrants, their different cultures and lifestyles, and by how quickly they were arriving and changing Israeli society. This sentiment was identified by visiting American journalist Irwin Shaw: "There is fear in Israel that the old, painfully formed codes of conduct and modes of life will be smothered by the massive immigration of Jews from the Diaspora."[14]

While all this was happening, as they emerged from the war and took on statehood and massive immigration, the newly independent Israelis had so much more to confront. They were establishing and crystallizing government bodies, implementing democratic rule, and trying to gain support on the global stage. They were trying to ensure that the various and often bitterly inimical Jewish fighting groups would now work as the unified Israel Defense Forces, when only a few months earlier, they had almost ended up in a civil war.[15] There was the context of the ongoing Arab-Israeli conflict that left many Israelis with the dreadful feeling that another major attack on the country was just a matter of time. In addition to the challenges of housing and health care, there were hard questions about religion and citizenship that had to be answered: What would be the place and boundaries of religion in a Jewish state? How would citizenship be determined? How was a Jew to be defined?[16] How would the Jewish state make a place for its non-Jewish minority?[17] And all these processes of state building, nation building, and self-definition were happening only just barely after the end of the Holocaust—that most profound catastrophe when, from 1933 to 1945, Jews "were robbed of their rights, dispossessed of their property, and slaughtered without pity."[18]

Across Israel, people had dire material needs. There was a severe nationwide economic shortage, a housing shortage, a shortage of food, and a shortage of other basic necessities such as clothes and shoes.[19] An official austerity policy began in 1949. Its aim was to "decrease consumption, increase production, and ensure that the entire population, including needy new immigrants, received the food and other goods they needed."[20] Although the austerity program was significantly reduced in 1953, it was officially cancelled only in 1959.[21] Under austerity, food supplies were rationed, and a heavy burden fell on homemakers across the country—especially housewives—who spent their days waiting in long, onerous lines for their meager food supplies while constantly struggling to care for their families.[22] Although, as Anat Helman and Orit Bashkin have shown, people often coped with these challenges with levity and humor, throughout much of the country, there was an atmosphere of hardship and scarcity.[23]

The housing crisis was directly connected to both the extreme economic shortage and the huge number of arriving immigrants. Although there were many challenges related to lodgings, the central experience of the housing crisis during the mass immigration is the Israeli transit camps for immigrants, called *ma'abarot*. These long-term but temporary settlements for new immigrants were introduced in 1950. Because nothing else was available, the "houses" were generally tents or tin huts. A powerful association was formed between transit camps and the mass immigration.

The infrastructure for immigrant absorption and settlement that Israel relied on when the country was established in May 1948 was based on what was already in place before statehood. Since the Jewish immigrants to Mandate Palestine in the 1940s had been given all-encompassing support from within the Jewish community, this was the framework for immigrant absorption in the 1950s.[24] Before 1948, new arrivals were temporarily housed in camps that "had one role—to act as a 'hostel' in preparation for moving to permanent settlements in the city or country."[25] Individuals did not need to pay for any of the services or the care they received in the immigrant camps. In May 1948, there were nine such camps throughout Israel—mostly in the center of the country—and more were eventually built, first in the center and then farther north. At the end of 1949, there were eighty-six thousand people in immigrant camps.[26] This system of housing Jewish newcomers in "immigrant houses" or "immigrant camps" changed in 1950 with the creation of the transit camps, which were established as an alternative framework meant to reduce dependency on state funded social services. The government plan was for immigrants to start being more independent and to also be less isolated from other Israelis. A main difference between the earlier model of immigrant camps and the later model of transit camps was jobs. Newcomers were meant to live in the transit camp but support themselves through work in nearby cities or agricultural settlements. Another important difference was a wider geographical distribution of the population. While the immigrant camps were mostly located in the center of the country, transit camps were dispersed throughout the entire country.[27]

The first transit camp opened in 1950. By the end of 1951, there were sixty-two, housing 220,517 people. As of 1952, they were slowly dismantled. The acute housing shortage ended in 1953 and interim places of residence—such as immigrant camps or transit camps—were done away with altogether.[28] The new immigrants were taken directly to their place of settlement immediately upon arrival in Israel.[29] At the end of 1963, eleven years after the dismantling of transit camps began, there were still 15,300 people living in these temporary settlements. People stayed for anywhere from one to eight years.[30] The extremely difficult experience of the transit camps is deeply imprinted on Israeli public memory and culture. They are remembered primarily as places of social isolation, hardship, and humiliation.[31]

Health was another one of Israel's major challenges and near crises in this time. There was widespread fear that the new country would be overwhelmed by more sick immigrants than it was equipped to care for and that dangerous epidemics would spread. Of the many grave challenges in this period, one of the reasons disease stands out is because good health was so central to what the Zionists had hoped to bring about in the Jewish state; there was a deep hope that they had left poor health and ailments behind in the Diaspora. In Zionist thought, Diasporic life had made the Jews physically and psychically diminished.[32] According to nineteenth-century Zionist thinker Max Nordau, Jews in the Diaspora had absorbed the degenerate qualities of the modern age. They had become urbane, superficial intellectuals, distanced from productive labor, with high-strung, nervous constitutions.[33] The hope among Zionists was that once the Jewish people returned to the land of Israel, both would be cured; if the Jews were allowed the opportunity to be industrious and active in physical labor, the land and all its inhabitants would prosper.[34] Nordau believed that the emergence of an athletic "muscle Jew" was necessary to restore health to the Jewish people in body and spirit.[35] Theodor Herzl brought this philosophy to life in *Altneuland*. In his canonical, utopian Zionist novel, after the Jews settle in the land of Israel, they are transformed from the sickly, frivolous, and ignoble characters of Europe into strong, well-built visions of health.[36]

With Zionist settlement to Palestine, these ideas were put into practice.[37] Science, technology, medicine, and public health were employed to help create the ideal Jewish state and help bring about the "healthy" transformation of the land and the people.[38] Early Zionist settlers to Palestine had arrived in a country with a rich medical marketplace, but they dreamed of more.[39] They eagerly pursued good health, incorporating European and American concepts of medicine and public health alongside Jewish traditions of caring for the sick, *bikur holim* and *linat tzedek*.[40] Jewish doctors, born and trained in Europe, were brought over by philanthropists Moses Montefiore and Baron Edmond de Rothschild as part of their settlement projects in the mid-nineteenth century.[41] Over time, more hospitals were opened and health insurance programs were established.[42] Parenting manuals were distributed among mothers to instruct them on how best to raise healthy Zionist children.[43] "Health Week" forums were held to educate the public on the benefits of physical activity, personal and public hygiene, and nutrition. The prestate Yishuv waged an ardent "war" on disease, most famously malaria, trachoma, and ringworm. They invested significant material, technological, and intellectual resources with the aim of spreading good health and ridding their community of illness.

By the time Shaar Ha'aliya was opened, the belief in the degenerate, sick Diaspora body was a deep-rooted, decades-old tradition. Although this was not always the reality, the popular self-image the Israelis perpetuated was of health and vigorous strength with a conviction of having left illness and weakness behind them in the Diaspora.[44] Yet as I will explore more deeply in chapter 2, a large percentage of the immigrants who arrived after 1948 were terribly sick. As such, the mass immigration put the Zionists in a position where they had to confront their own demons.[45] Arriving on their shores in the thousands were flesh-and-blood reminders of the reality that they were trying to distance themselves from: that the "weak" and "diminished" Diaspora Jew is an indissoluble part of the "strong" and "healthy" Israeli and that disease and contagion would be an inevitable, challenging, and—at times—polarizing part of the new state.

With the Holocaust just barely behind them, the war of independence only just won, and the new state being cobbled together, this was a time that was intensely vulnerable for Jewish Israelis; it was filled with deep anxiety regarding what the future would bring. This environment of uncertainty, instability, and seismic change was the setting for mass immigration. As Irwin Shaw put it, immigration was only one "huge, dark puzzle for a nation rich in puzzles."[46] One of the ways that this "dark puzzle" was approached in the 1950s was through the state's official "melting pot" absorption policy. Education, medicine, language, military participation, religious practice, and culture were all used to transform the immigrants from Diaspora Jews with different backgrounds into a unified nation.[47] But the term *melting pot* is a misnomer that wrongly conveys equity. In fact, the policy, as beautifully described by Henrietta Dahan-Khalev, was often a painful and repressive one of "Ashkenazi-ization." As an immigrant child from Morocco, Dahan-Khalev was taught, "All that is Mizrakhi is retarded, degenerate, and primitive." She describes the melting pot experience as "an educational, intellectual, and economic steam roller that squashed everything and left no room for any self-development outside of that of a distorting Ashkenazi, Zionist, Israeli, and European hegemony."[48] The isolated area of Shaar Ha'aliya was the first stop in the melting pot process. A Jewish Agency report outlined its two main aims: "How to turn the new immigrant into a citizen of Israel in only a few days, and how to protect the Yishuv from diseases."[49] It was more than just a place where new immigrants would spend a few days to undergo basic processing, it was an isolated space where people were meant to leave behind their Diasporic "ailments" before crossing the border into Israel.

Facing Shaar Ha'aliya, 1949–1962

Arrival

Immigrants arrived at Shaar Ha'aliya after reaching Israel on ships at the
Haifa port or on planes at the Lod airport. From there, they would get onto
a truck that would drive them to the camp. Shaar Ha'aliya was situated
near the Haifa shore, right next to a beautiful view of the Mediterranean
Sea. The camp itself was huge. It was built to hold five thousand people
and had administrative buildings, hundreds of cabins, medical facilities,
synagogues, and dining halls. When the immigrants arrived, their first
stop in the camp would be the reception desk where their name and personal information would be recorded for the camp's statistical department.
At this point, they would be given a personal card, a document on which the
various camp departments would record information throughout their
stay.[50] Next, they might receive a document explaining, in Hebrew, what
to expect in Shaar Ha'aliya: "New Immigrant. Welcome to Shaar Ha'aliya.
You have been sent here with the express purpose of undergoing the medical examination [. . .] Do not request an exit permit. Exiting is forbidden
until you leave here in a couple of days. To where? Family, a kibbutz or a
transit camp. This will be determined after you undergo the final medical
exam."[51] Registration took place whenever boats arrived: in the middle of
the night, early in the morning, in the afternoon heat, on the Sabbath, and
even religious or national holidays.[52] The policy and intention was that the
immigrants would be greeted with food and drink; sometimes this was
possible, and sometimes it was not.[53] At registration the new arrival would
be lent equipment that they would need for the duration of their stay at
Shaar Ha'aliya: a mattress, a sheet and blanket, a lantern, a fork and spoon,
a plate and mug. Then it would be time to find and get settled in the camp
lodgings.[54]

Where a person slept would depend on how crowded the camp was at
the time of their arrival. Although things had been carefully planned, any
hope for an efficiently running system quickly fell through very soon after

the camp opened.[55] The enormous rate of immigration was overwhelming, and it became impossible to evacuate the immigrants already staying
there before new ships arrived. Some people did complete their processing
and leave the camp in a number of days, but many others ended up staying in Shaar Ha'aliya for weeks or months at a time. Because of language
and general miscommunication, people did not always understand where
they were supposed to be and when. They missed compulsory appointments and had to wait for another day before they could leave the camp.
Others refused to leave until they were given the housing assignments in
Israel that they wanted.[56] Very soon after it opened, the camp overflowed
with people.[57] It was built to accommodate no more than five thousand,
but at its peak, it housed ten to twelve thousand. So depending on when
a person arrived, the possibilities for where they would stay were cabins,
tents, or any other haphazard arrangements when there was nothing else
available.[58] One family was housed in the police cabin when nothing
else could be found.[59] Another woman spent her first night at Shaar
Ha'aliya outside, sleeping on her luggage.[60]

Each cabin held around thirty beds.[61] Conditions in the tents and cabins
were notoriously poor. They were dirty, tents collapsed in winter storms,
dirt floors turned to mud, and people and their belongings were soaked.[62]
Sometimes there were makeshift dividers, like sheets or blankets, to create
a semblance of privacy.[63] In some cases, a person would have shared lodgings with others of the same background or, at least, people who shared
a common language. But someone might also end up in the tent or cabin
with people who were completely foreign, with no common language to be
able to break barriers and initiate contact. The people who went through
Shaar Ha'aliya came from all the immigration countries in Israel of those
years. The largest communities to go through Shaar Ha'aliya were from
Iraq, Romania, Poland, Turkey, and Iran. There were North African immigrants from Egypt, Libya, Tunisia, Algeria, and Morocco.[64] One log entry
from 1954 lists twenty-seven different countries that were represented in
the camp over a period of six months with places as diverse as China,

Belgium, Morocco, Austria, Spain, Persia, France, and Yemen.[65] The waves of migration through Shaar Ha'aliya naturally corresponded with the national waves of immigration. The Polish and North African immigrants arrived largely in 1949 and 1950. Then there was a new wave of Moroccan immigration after 1955. The largest waves of Iraqi and Romanian immigration took place at the same time, in 1950–1951.[66]

The fact that there was foreignness and a lack of a common language doesn't necessarily mean that there was no kindness and intimacy. The stories of immigrants in Israel during the 1950s are so full of accounts of the kindness of strangers and general acts of human goodness that one can assume that in the Shaar Ha'aliya tents and cabins, there were day-to-day acts of warmth to put one another at ease. In this way, the discomfort caused by the lack of privacy could have been at least partially relieved. But for another person, the scenario could have been very different. Reports indicate cases of violence, prostitution, and theft. There were people who intimidated and attacked their peers.[67] And so the shared living space could have been not only just uncomfortable but genuinely frightening if someone had to sleep unguarded next to potentially threatening strangers.

Waiting in Line

When it came time to eat, the immigrant would go to get food from a central kitchen and dining hall. They had a separate food card glued to their personal card that was stamped for every meal. Once all meals had been stamped, the food card was torn off and the immigrant had to go to the camp office to arrange for a new meal card.[68] The plan was that all meals would be consumed in the hall. In practice, families would usually send a representative who would bring back the food rations to the living quarters.[69] While the original intention was that the immigrants and the staff would eat together, by June 1949, a separate dining hall was opened for the staff, with the explanation that the number of immigrants had grown so significantly that there was a problem with space.[70] Special effort was put into ensuring that the entire premises were kosher. The food that

was given in the camp was simple and limited, in keeping with the austerity guidelines in the country at the time. There was bread, margarine, soft
cheeses, eggs, fish, olives, vegetables, and jam.[71]

It would have been impossible for these foods to be satisfying or pleas-
ing to all people from such different culinary traditions. Immigrants
complained about the food and much was thrown away. As a result, the
food at Shaar Ha'aliya remained a very central part of the memory of
the immigrants who had been there.[72] But food also had other significance,
as a tool for state policy. In 1950, when overcrowding became a major problem, a policy was introduced where immigrants who refused to leave Shaar
Ha'aliya for their permanent places of residence would not get food.[73] This
measure was initiated as a way to solve the issue of overcrowding in the
camp by forcing people out. It also shows a shift in the country's absorption policy to try to decrease the immigrant's dependence on state funds.

The way this system worked was that when people arrived at Shaar
Ha'aliya they would be given only the number of coupons that would
bring them to the time of their medical examination. The remaining coupons were contingent on appearing for the examination.[74] If, for health
reasons, a person were instructed to stay on in Shaar Ha'aliya, they would
be given additional coupons. If not, they were given only coupons to last
until they were scheduled to leave the camp—up to three days. If anyone refused to leave on the scheduled day, they were no longer eligible to
receive food in the camp.

In these various ways, food played a significant role in the immigrant's experience at Shaar Ha'aliya. While it does show the new, poor
state providing for its immigrants, it also shows the state using the denial
of nourishment as a mechanism for control. The eating environment at
Shaar Ha'aliya shows the immigrant seeking out the family unit, rejecting
the common dining hall for the family tent. The food itself symbolized the
newness and foreignness of the immigrant's experience, as the sensual
pleasure of eating, the comforting act of consuming familiar tastes and
textures, became unappealing or strange.

Yet before anyone was able to get to the food in the dining hall, they would have to wait in line. One photograph of Shaar Ha'aliya shows at least fifty-eight people in line and another has more than one hundred—and these are only the people visible to the camera.[75] Meal times were not the only occasions where the immigrants had to deal with long, crowded lines. There are accounts of long lines for the medical examinations and for the final processing committee.[76] Journalists mentioned them in articles, employees referred to them in reports, and immigrants complained about them in letters. The grueling line became a symbol of Shaar Ha'aliya.

These lines resulted from overcrowding, misunderstandings, poor communication, and eagerness to leave Shaar Ha'aliya as soon as possible. Because of language barriers, people did not always understand where they were supposed to be and when. Sometimes people would arrive at their appointments early—because they were eager to finish the processing as quickly as possible and leave the camp—and they would end up waiting for hours. Lines were an inextricable part of the immigrant's experience at Shaar Ha'aliya. They were a place where people interacted with one another. They could last for hours. They were numerous and tedious and they wore people down as they waited indeterminately. Though they eventually ended, it was at the end of the waiting that the new immigrant, often exhausted and frustrated, interacted with the Shaar Ha'aliya staff and processing bodies.

Work

Many of the employees were themselves immigrants, with varying degrees of newness. There were health care workers, office administrators, kitchen staff, as well as police officers. It is not clear exactly how many people were employed at Shaar Ha'aliya, but it would appear that the largest count, in 1950, was around four hundred, when the number of immigrants at the camp was at its peak.[77] Work at Shaar Ha'aliya was a complicated mixture of myth and reality. On the one hand, it gave the employee a certain sense of honor because it was an opportunity for the individual to take part in the Zionist mission of Jewish immigration to the land of Israel. From a practical perspective, it provided the security of a paying job with vacation time and opportunities for promotion during the difficult economy of Israel's first years. On the other hand, the work at Shaar Ha'aliya was very difficult. The camp was isolated, attendance was required at 7 a.m. and arriving to work even ten minutes late meant losing an entire day's salary.[78]

What made the work even more challenging was the camp's cramped, uncomfortable environment. The staff who worked there were under extreme pressure.[79] In many cases, there wasn't a common language between the immigrants and the camp personnel, and often there seemed to be no way to bridge the huge cultural gaps that separated people. Inevitably, there was tension between the staff members, between the staff and the director, and of course, between the staff and the hundreds of immigrants arriving at the camp nearly every day.

Health services in the camp were overseen by the government and the Jewish Agency's Immigrant Health Services as well as Kupat Holim Clalit, the largest and most powerful sick fund at the time.[80] The main aim of the health care services was to determine who would require treatment for infectious diseases and who would require hospitalization. During medical examinations, doctors were looking for signs of ringworm and trachoma, blood samples were drawn to test for syphilis and gonorrhea, and minograph exams were conducted to identify tuberculosis.[81] The minograph, a small photo-roentgenography machine that was much cheaper and quicker than getting X-rays, was used to conduct the preliminary chest examinations.[82] Large X-rays were then ordered in a smaller number of cases when the minograph came out suspect.[83] If your minograph did not show any signs of tuberculosis, you would be vaccinated with BCG.

Additional medical services located on the Shaar Ha'aliya premises included a mother-infant care center (*tipat halav*) as well as a hospital and isolation building. In 1952, a large center for treatment of children with ringworm and trachoma was opened in a fenced-off section of the camp.[84]

Except for this institute, Shaar Ha'aliya was not intended as a location for long-term care. However, in contrast to situations like those in Ellis Island, for example, medicine did not act as a gatekeeper that weeded out immigrants for deportation. At Shaar Ha'aliya, medical examinations were meant to identify cases of disease that would then be treated in various health care facilities throughout the country.

THE RINGWORM AND TRACHOMA INSTITUTE, SHAAR HA'ALIYA, 1952–1960

There were, however, two diseases that were targeted for treatment right on the Shaar Ha'aliya premises. In January 1952, the Jewish Agency opened the Shaar Ha'aliya Institute for the Treatment of Ringworm and Trachoma, Israel's central health care facility of this nature for immigrant children.[85] Here, thousands of children received medical attention as part of their immigration process, and (as will be discussed further in chapter 4) its story—particularly because of ringworm treatment—is at the heart of an ongoing saga of trauma and controversy in contemporary Israel.

Trachoma is a highly contagious bacterial infection of the eyes. In the early twentieth century, it was one of the leading causes of acquired blindness, particularly among children.[86] Ringworm of the scalp, or *Tinea capitis*, is a fungal infection that also primarily affects children. It tends to appear on a person's head as hairless, shiny, greasy-looking patches. By the 1840s, ringworm was identified as a fungal disease caused by various tinea species.[87] It almost always occurs before the age of fifteen, spontaneously clearing by puberty.[88] And although it is highly contagious, it poses no physical danger.

As carriers of very visible, contagious diseases, trachoma and ringworm patients have long been ostracized and stigmatized throughout the world.[89] For example, in the early twentieth century, immigrants with ringworm or trachoma were denied entry into the United States (trachoma was listed under the category of "dangerous" contagious diseases, while ringworm was listed as a "loathsome" disease).[90] In the Israeli establishment of 1952, you see a continuation of this stigmatization; they were framed as the ailments of people seen as impoverished, backward, and dirty.

The decision to open the separate ringworm and trachoma institute on the Shaar Ha'aliya premises was directly tied to the selective immigration policy:[91] "Barring the immigration of those sick with one of those two diseases would bring the immigration from North Africa to a halt, for there the diseases are so common that there is almost not a single family that is not infected."[92] Since ringworm and trachoma were both so prevalent as well as curable over a relatively short period of time, the Ministry of Health and the Jewish Agency's Absorption Department reached an agreement: instead of barring the entry of these children, they would open a center in Israel where, immediately upon arrival, they would receive treatment for these diseases. The southern section of the Shaar Ha'aliya camp was the chosen location, on a plot of land that had already been earmarked for a general health care center for the treatment of young immigrants.[93]

In December 1951, Dr. Chaim Sheba (then deputy director-general of the Ministry of Health) wrote to Israeli health care representatives in France by way of the Jewish philanthropic organization OSE (*Oeuvre de Secours aux Enfants*): "We are prepared to receive, every month, 100–150 cases of ringworm and treat them in Israel. Dr. Josephtal has agreed for them to be concentrated in Shaar Ha'aliya."[94] Sheba's plan was that, in time, these people would eventually become a productive part of the workforce: "While it seems that we are bringing in the sick, we are actually saving the Israeli nation a lot of money, and it may be that you can find other types that right now are an economic and moral burden, and you may in fact find that it is precisely the institutions in Israel that get them back into a state fit for work. So, of course you will be bringing people who are apparently sick . . . but you will still be easing the State of Israel's burden, from an economic standpoint."[95] Although the initial plan for the center, as outlined by Chaim Sheba, was to focus on ringworm, it evolved into a place where trachoma would also be treated, since there were many children who also had trachoma or who had both diseases. Additionally, various documents attest to the fact that the camp also gave medical care to youth with sexually transmitted diseases.[96] From the time that it opened in 1952 until the time it closed in 1960, around twelve thousand children were treated at Shaar Ha'aliya's Ringworm and Trachoma Institute.[97]

The actual place was built for up to five hundred children and had a staff of twenty to thirty individuals.[98] It was made up of "dormitories, shower-rooms for patients and staff, offices and a barber-shop."[99] There was also a sports field and a social hall.[100] Children were meant to be isolated in the center until the end of their treatment—from a month to three months for ringworm and around two months for trachoma.[101] This isolation was not easy. On Israel's independence day the children were forced to watch the parade while sitting inside cars, away from the others.[102] There was a Purim holiday where the only people the children were allowed to have come and celebrate with them were the Jewish Agency representatives and health care workers.[103] But it would seem that by Passover of 1955, those stringent rules had been at least partially relaxed and the majority of the children from the institute were given permission to go and celebrate the holiday with their families in towns and immigrant transit camps.[104]

The purpose of the center went beyond the purely clinical—it was envisioned and operated as a "medical-educational institute."[105] In the letter from 1951 that outlined the plan to found the institute, Dr. Chaim Sheba defended its establishment as a way to "productivize" new immigrants and turn them from the infirm into able-bodied citizens capable of contributing to the economy.[106] Numerous documents refer to the educational dimension of life in the camp, including agricultural training, to promote a love of the land and pioneering skills; a cultural program with crafts, song, and dance; as well as Hebrew language lessons: "For the duration of the two months that every child had to stay in the camp until the end of treatment, he acquires for himself a knowledge of the language and the land as well as habits for working the land—which in future will turn into a love of the land—the homeland."[107] This combination of medicine and education became a way to influence the process through which the children would become ideal Israeli citizens: healthy, Hebrew-speaking pioneers. Indeed, the ringworm and trachoma institute was said to have two aims: "Healing the body and spiritual preparation for life in Israel."[108,109]

Photographs of trachoma patients at Shaar Ha'aliya show children in a line waiting for their turn with a nurse who is administering drops.[110] These children received their treatment several times throughout the morning over a period of around twenty-seven days.[111] In these photographs the children do not look very happy, but the experience is not often referred to in documents on Shaar Ha'aliya or recalled in oral testimony—a fact that suggests that the medical treatment for trachoma was largely felt to be unremarkable. This is hardly the case for ringworm.

The treatment for ringworm given in Shaar Ha'aliya, as in other ringworm facilities in Israel during that period, was the Adamson-Kienbock technique. This accepted, biomedical remedy of its day was severe. It included shaving the child's hair, waxing the head, and applying irradiation.[112] Originally, children in the institute had been taken to Haifa for radiation treatment as a temporary arrangement until Shaar Ha'aliya became equipped with X-ray machines. Eventually, Shaar Ha'aliya acquired three X-ray machines for the ringworm patients.[113]

From the perspective of the children, this medical treatment was awful. It was extremely painful, aggressive, invasive, and scarring:

> They shaved my head, held me forcibly, and spread some glue on my head . . . She pulled my hair by force, and actually scalped me . . . After plucking out my hair she held me like this [demonstrates] between her legs. She grabbed my head between her knees and plucked with the tweezers like I was a chicken. If I'd dare to move I'd get a what for . . . I

was laid down on a table and tied up like a lamb . . . and then I remember some round contraption being put on my head . . . like an old fash-
ioned hair drier, and it felt like electrical stings.[114]

Three nurses who worked in the ringworm and trachoma center retained
similarly harsh memories of the medical treatment. They recall trying to
comfort crying, distraught children while actually feeling that what the
children were going through was "awful" and "traumatic."[115]

For the young patients, a factor that made the trauma of the treatment
even worse was that it left them bald. A woman who immigrated from
Morocco in 1953 recalls how humiliating it was for her—as a young, devel-
oping, eleven-year-old girl—to have no hair: "We always went around
with a head-covering and we wouldn't take it off. The moment we would
take them off they would say to us: 'Hey. You have a light bulb on your
head. You aren't human beings.' They were simply . . . you know there were
children who were very cruel . . . very . . . other children who hadn't had it
done to them . . . and it continued and continued."[116] The misery that the
children experienced because they were bald was captured by the Israeli
novelist Eli Amir in his novel *Scapegoat*. In a conversation between two
boys—both immigrants from Iraq—Nuri, the novel's protagonist, learns
the reason for the head-coverings that were so popular among the immigrant children:

"You all get a crew cut?" I asked.
    "Even the girls," he replied.
    "What?" A broken cry escaped my mouth. "The girls? Poor things!"
    "Ya'allah with this life." Now I understood the meaning of all the
head-coverings.
    "Lice, flies, plague, leprosy, ringworm, shmingworm . . ." singsonged
the boy, Reuven.
    "Enough!" I screamed.
    "Let them go to hell. In Baghdad my mother worked in the commu-
nity's clinic. Doesn't understand why the baldness," he said.[117]

This dialogue shows the despair caused by the shaved heads, the perceived link between the immigrants and disease as well as the immigrants' skepticism of the health care treatment given to them in their new home. One woman poignantly captures the injury caused by the ringworm treatment: "Why did they do that to me? I had beautiful curls, why did they do it?"[118]

Despite the obvious distress caused to the children from this unattractive physical appearance, marking them as foreign and contagious, it has been asked whether the stigma would have been any less if, instead of the baldness, the children had been left with traces of ringworm—also a very visible stigma.[119] As mentioned earlier, ringworm of the scalp was categorized as a "loathsome contagious disease."[120] That is to say that ringworm was considered so repugnant that the mere sight of it, and the threat of its being transmitted, made it "loathed" the world over—even when it was known to be not actually dangerous. The repellent power of this disease has shaped what Charles Rosenberg has referred to as "the total experience of sickness."[121] Ringworm victims have had a painful "total experience" throughout history.

The treatment method used at Shaar Ha'aliya—a central point in the Israeli controversy—was not an Israeli invention; under the guidance of global health organizations, standard, international medical procedures were adopted. Moreover, the Shaar Ha'aliya Institute was not the only facility in Israel that treated people with ringworm and trachoma.[122] Its significance lies in its focus on new immigrants, primarily immigrants from North Africa and the Middle East. The children treated at Shaar Ha'aliya were all newcomers—either immigrants whose families had passed through Shaar Ha'aliya or immigrant children from the transit camps.[123] These children were taken from their families and brought to Shaar Ha'aliya for the period of treatment. There is also evidence that the Ministry of Health had wanted Arab children with ringworm and trachoma to be treated at Shaar Ha'aliya as well, but because of a lack of space, this request could not be honored.[124] No similar request could be found for Jewish children born in Israel. This fact raises important issues. Use of the ringworm and trachoma center was not determined by geographical accessibility; immigrant children from all over the country, including the then remote southern region, were brought there for treatment. Thus the decision not to have Israeli-born *sabra* children treated there could not be explained by practical, logistical considerations. The idea that the Shaar Ha'aliya Ringworm and Trachoma Institute was conceived for only immigrant and Arab children signifies its conceptual role as an isolated space for marginalized social groups: immigrant children primarily from Arab countries as well as Arab children who were citizens of Israel.

The fact that the Shaar Ha'aliya Institute focused on immigrant children meant that the trauma from the illness and the treatment procedure exacerbated the trauma of immigration. Parents and children were often separated from one another immediately after they had just arrived in the new and foreign country. The separation, which lasted up to several months, was very severe. In many cases, the parents lived in towns that were hours away and Shaar Ha'aliya was difficult to access by what was then an underdeveloped public transportation system. Few, if any, would have had access to private vehicles. Although there were some telephones at Shaar Ha'aliya, their use was very limited, and there is no indication that the children and their parents could have been in contact by phone. This rupture to the newly displaced family unit was traumatic for children and parents alike. The administrators' and the caregivers' approach to the children at the Shaar Ha'aliya Institute was not intentionally malicious. Nevertheless, the physical and emotional harshness of the treatment method for so minor a skin condition are an important reminder of how misguided and detrimental biomedicine can be.

SHAAR HA'ALIYA BET

In 1951, the same year that the plan for the Ringworm and Trachoma Institute was finalized, the crowding at Shaar Ha'aliya became intolerable and a temporary camp was opened to help reduce the number of people at the main camp. This camp, called Shaar Ha'aliya Bet (literally, Shaar Ha'aliya "B"), remained open through part of 1952. It was located close to Haifa, in Atlit, in what had formerly been the British detention center for illegal Jewish immigrants.[125] By 1952, the population of Shaar Ha'aliya was significantly reduced, the combined result of the change in immigration policy (selective immigration was introduced in November 1951) and the declining number of immigrants to Israel. Slowly, tents were brought down, staff laid off, and buildings closed. In 1955, only several hundred immigrants went through Shaar Ha'aliya, as opposed to the tens of thousands of previous years.[126] The number of staff was similarly reduced, so that by March 1955, Shaar Ha'aliya had only twenty-six staff members, excluding the ringworm and trachoma center.[127] In these later years, the only immigrants brought to the camp were those who the Jewish Agency considered "problem cases" in terms of processing, such as people with disabilities and elderly individuals who did not have family to care for them.[128]

Shaar Ha'aliya was officially closed in 1962 after slowly petering out. On one of the last days before it was dismantled, Yehuda Weisberger went to Shaar Ha'aliya with a journalist and two former colleagues. The camp stood uninhabited, a relic from a different time. The three men reminisced as they walked in the emptied space, through deserted huts and offices and quiet pathways. Thirteen years had passed since the camp had opened, since the day Yehuda and Leah Weisberger posed solemnly for the photograph by the Shaar Ha'aliya sign, documenting its opening. Now a middle-aged man, a father of two children, the camp had given Yehuda much to remember as he walked through the hollowed-out premises. He had been a part of an extraordinary chapter in the founding of the Jewish state, one that imprinted the lives of nearly half a million people, and he looked around with pride and regret. After the men finished their stroll, bulldozers would come through to reclaim the landscape. They would pull down the cabins, flatten the buildings, dismantle the fence. And with that, Israel's "gate of immigration" was finally closed.[129]

CHAPTER 2

Structure

Sylvia Meltzer was a child when she moved to Israel. "It was like a dream come true," she recalls. Life in Romania had become "uncomfortable and unpleasant" for Sylvia and her family after their store was taken from them and they were left with no income. The only way for her father to survive would have been to fake loyalty to the Communist government. "So for us," she remembers, immigration was "a good experience."

When they arrived in Israel, Sylvia's parents were delayed at Shaar Ha'aliya for several months because her younger sister was sick and they needed to stay with her while she recovered. Sylvia, however, left Shaar Ha'aliya almost immediately. She went home with an aunt who was already settled in the country and who had decided to take her under her wing; but, even while she lived with her aunt, Sylvia returned to Shaar Ha'aliya regularly to spend time with her family. Years after her arrival in Israel, she was interviewed about her immigration experience. This is how she describes going to visit her parents in Shaar Ha'aliya:

SYLVIA: [...] when I went to visit I would go out through a hole in the
    fence, because I don't think they let people go out.
INTERVIEWER: Where would you go from the hole in the fence? This
    was because you wanted to go where? To Haifa?

SYLVIA: I would go to my aunt's. I would go visit my parents and then
   return to my aunt.

INTERVIEWER: And you remember that all this was done through a
   hole in the fence?

SYLVIA: Yes. Maybe we were just too lazy to go [through] the gate.

At this point in the interview, Sylvia's husband, Eliezer, adds the following:

ELIEZER: No, no. My uncle used to go in through the hole in the fence,
   where the gas station is today. We used to leave from there, we got
   on a bus and went to Tel Aviv.

SYLVIA: I always entered and exited through a hole in the fence. I
   remember that clearly.[1]

An essential element to a quarantine is a physical barrier. The physical
barrier at Shaar Ha'aliya, the barbed wire fence, was meant to contain
the contagious diseases the immigrants might have been carrying. Yet it
was not only a structure of confinement but also a site of movement and
a vehicle for defiance. As seen in the Capa photograph and as described
by Sylvia Meltzer, this was a negotiable barrier for the many immigrants
who crossed it with relative ease; but the police, who were responsible for
enforcing the quarantine, were upset by the way these breaches under-
mined their authority and frustrated their attempts at keeping order. As
a result, they pushed to have the fence reinforced. These struggles surrounding the structure were not simply about whether it would be open
or closed but rather about whether the balance of power would favor those
who wanted Shaar Ha'aliya to be isolated by a fence or those who rebelled
against it.

   And so while this is a story about a physical structure and the negotiation of its boundaries, it is also a story about how power was negotiated
between new immigrants and the new Israel. The state agents tried to use a
quarantine as a way to control the immigrants' arrival and integration, and

(as will be discussed in chapter 3) they relied heavily on the threat of disease as a way to understand and justify the quarantine; but the immigrants rather easily and naturally rebelled against this containment. The defiance of the fence was part of a larger context of immigrant rebellion and protest in Shaar Ha'aliya. Thus despite their new immigrant status and the harsh conditions at the camp, the people arriving at and staying in Shaar Ha'aliya were quickly and significantly empowered when up against the authority of the state and its various mechanisms of power, including, but not exclusive to, health care.

STRUCTURES OF QUARANTINE

By using a fence, later reinforced with police officers, to buttress a medically defended isolation, Israel was doing something that was not at all new. Quarantine is an ancient and cross-cultural phenomenon that does not look any one, defined way. In its various incarnations over time and place, you can find vastly different structures, with vastly different methods and severity of enforcement that, despite the differences, have been defined as quarantines.

The biblical discussion of isolation for lepers in Leviticus 13 is largely understood as the starting point for the European concept of quarantine; but this passage does not describe what the quarantine, or isolation, looked like. Instead, it emphasizes the distance put between the community and the "contaminated" person: "He shall be unclean as long as the disease is on him. Being unclean, he shall dwell apart; his dwelling shall be outside the camp."[2] In Leviticus, there is a distinction between isolation and dwelling apart. These words appear in the original Hebrew as: הסגיר (hisgir—isolate) and בדד (badad—alone, or dwell apart). *Hisgir* is the source for the modern Hebrew word for quarantine, הסגר (hesger), while *badad* is the more severe term *alone*. Isolation is a time in which the disease undergoes surveillance, to see how it will develop. Dwelling apart is what follows when isolation has failed. It is the fate of the unclean *metzora*, or leper. To return to the community after dwelling apart, the priest must guide the person through a meticulous cleansing ritual, only at the end of which "he shall be clean."[3]

Historian James A. Diamond writes that in the rabbinic tradition this separation is alternately understood as curative and punitive. The separation was a harsh decree, carrying with it a stigma and the hardship of being alone, but it was also an opportunity to be healed and purified. This biblical idea of quarantine places the emphasis on the individual—by being secluded, a person would have a chance to heal. It perhaps then follows that the community would also benefit by having the "unclean" person out of its midst, but the biblical text does not make this explicit. In contrast to more modern conceptions of quarantine in which the health of the group is the main theme, the Bible focuses on the individual's health and the broader community is not mentioned.[4]

In medieval Christendom, the enactments against lepers that appear in the Bible were further restricted, and a severe system of surveillance and ostracism was put into place. In this time, isolation became much more prohibitive and more clearly and forcefully structured. George Rosen refers to medieval lepers as "the living dead." They were outcast from the community for their entire lives, stripped of civic rights, and "considered dead socially long before receiving the merciful boon of physical death."[5] This approach to lepers later provided the framework on which the European concept of state-supervised quarantine was instituted. When the great pandemic of plague broke out in the fourteenth century, there was a basic comprehension that the plague was communicable. This fact, joined with the panic instilled by the acute fear of this very visibly horrifying disease, reinforced the desire to withdraw from people who were sick. Moreover, deeply entrenched Judeo-Christian traditions linked illness to sin and spiritual impurity. This is what ensued:

> Patients had to be reported to the authorities. They were then examined and isolated in their houses for the duration of the illness. Every house

containing a plague victim was placed under a ban. All who had come into contact with the patient were compelled to remain in isolation. Food and other necessities were provided by the municipal authorities through special messengers. The dead were passed through the windows and removed from the city in carts. Burial outside the city was likewise intended to prevent extension of the epidemic. When a plague patient died, the rooms were aired and fumigated, and the effects of the deceased were burned.[6]

It was in this environment of plague-ridden, fourteenth-century Italy that civic-supervised quarantine was first introduced: "A system of sanitary control to combat contagious diseases, with observation stations, isolation hospitals and disinfection procedures." The word quarantine was coined at this time. A forty-day period of isolation was enforced on both people and objects entering a port so that any symptoms of poor health could be observed, and in this way, the plague could be prevented from entering the city. The English word *quarantine* is derived from the Italian word for "forty": *quaranta.*[7]

Accounts from Native American cultures describe how different structures, from houses to entire villages, were turned into quarantines. In the eighteenth century, members of the Cherokee tribes would refuse to enter towns that were known to be affected by a smallpox epidemic. In some instances, severe steps were taken to make sure that nobody could leave quarantined areas. During an epidemic that broke out in 1748 in the Four Nations Upper Creek towns, communication with infected villages was terminated, sentinels were put on watch, and orders were given to kill anyone advancing from infected villages.[8] In addition to sealing off villages (a measure that historian Paul Kelton suggests might have been learned from the English) the First Nations practiced avoidance ceremonies in which the village was shut off from the outside world for an extended period as cleansing rituals were enacted.[9] In other cases, sick people were removed from their villages and were forbidden from having contact with other members of their tribe, not unlike the biblical lepers who were sent to "dwell apart."[10,11]

There was not as strict an incarceration of lepers in Muslim culture as there was in medieval Europe, but there were cases of separation. During the Islamic era in North Africa (excluding Egypt) and southern Spain, lepers were built special living quarters outside city walls.[12] A description written by a traveler in the mid-eighteenth century documents cases of forced isolation: "At Basra, lepers are shut up in a house by themselves; and there is a quarter in Baghdad surrounded with walls, and full of barracks, to which lepers are carried by force, if they retire not thither voluntarily."[13] In medieval Muslim countries, there were also cases in which people with syphilis were housed with the lepers outside of the city quarters.[14]

These Islamic traditions of quarantine and contagion first developed in response to the bubonic plague. Muhammad gave his followers instructions on how to deal specifically with plague as well as more general approaches to health and disease. These directives stemmed from his own experiences living through the first plague pandemics (541–750 CE), which hit the Mediterranean basin, parts of Europe, and the British Isles and predated the Black Death by eight centuries.[15] Muhammad's basic teachings raised a possibility that quarantine would be allowed by saying that "one should neither enter into nor seek to leave a place stricken by plague."[16] Scholars have noted that this recommendation seems to contradict Muhammad's teachings on the role of God in illness, but it is in fact similar to the common premodern approach, which straddles a rejection of notions of contagion while incorporating observations that disease is spread through contact.[17] Through plague, God was directly intervening in people's lives: faithful followers of Islam who were struck by the terrible illness were receiving an act of mercy that would bring them to martyrdom and Paradise; infidels who rejected Islam were receiving a just punishment for faithlessness and sin. This traditional Islamic approach, Joseph Byrne explains, "accepted both God's will and miasma as causes of plague, and the religion specifically taught that there was no contagion."[18]

Thus Islamic tradition left room for occasional implementation of quarantine but because of the emphasis on God's divine role in disease, the encounter with plague in Muslim urban centers was met with "a level of acceptance and, perhaps, resignation that was quite different from that of Christian cities."[19]

The move from premodern traditions of contagion to the modern, scientifically driven contagionist theory is marked by Robert Koch's discovery of the tubercle bacillus in 1882. Dorothy Porter explains that this discovery brought about a "shift in emphasis [...] from the environment to the individual as the vector of transmission."[20] Thus the concept of quarantine, which had been derived out of an assumption that diseases were contagious, was now given the legitimacy of scientific authority.[21] Fear of disease became more directly focused on the people who were sick and who were then perceived as the public's victimizers. Eugenia Tognotti has described the important changes that shaped this later history: "A turning point in the history of quarantine came after the pathogenic agents of the most feared epidemic diseases were identified between the nineteenth and twentieth centuries."[22] In the years following Alexander Fleming's identification of penicillin in 1928, there was a "long anticipated therapeutic revolution,"[23] which eventually led to an increased certainty that scientific medicine had the power to fully defeat epidemic disease: "Reflecting the same sense of confidence in the *Pax antibiotica*, the U.S. surgeon general announced in 1969 that 'it was time to close the book on infectious diseases' because they no longer represented a serious threat to America's health."[24] This, of course, was not to be, as seen in the epidemics of the late twentieth and early twenty-first centuries, the diminished power of antibiotics in the face of drug resistant bacteria and the continued relevance of quarantine in the containment of disease.[25]

There are different qualities to the various incarnations of quarantine and protoquarantine. Some have an individual being removed from the group. There are other cases in which an entire group is enclosed and others refuse to approach it. Finally, there is the active flight whereby the people who are sick are abandoned by the healthy. The difference can be found in the action of the movement: whether the ill are made to leave, whether the healthy leave the ill, or whether the ill are in a group, sealed in and left unapproached by others. These different separations would also mean different fates. One would mean giving the person a time to heal; another meant a period of observation (allowing people to prove their good health); another meant leaving the sick to die, while yet another meant dooming the fate of the healthy by sealing them in to share the fate of the ill. Inevitably, there is someone declaring the person ill; there are the "healthy" who, in their presence, help define illness; and there is always some form of isolation.

Today there is an important medical distinction between quarantine and isolation. Isolation is the separation of someone who is known to have a communicable disease and who is thus kept isolated to prevent the spread of infection. Quarantine is the time in which someone who has potentially been exposed to a communicable disease is left isolated for a period of observation (much like the immigrants at Shaar Ha'aliya) to see whether the symptoms of the disease do indeed develop.[26] In some cases, quarantine is imposed so as to protect a person who is already sick, to protect a weak immune system from the hazards of other infection. There is no one physical form of a quarantine. It could be an island, a building, a hospital, or a village, or it could be a camp enclosed by a fence.

Contagion at Shaar Ha'aliya

Shaar Ha'aliya was built on the foundations of the former British army camp St. Luke's.[27] This meant that much of the infrastructure for the processing camp was already there before Shaar Ha'aliya even opened. Still, significant renovations were needed to adapt the premises to its new purpose of accommodating the thousands of immigrants who were expected to arrive. And so, over an intense ten weeks of renovations, the existing water, sewage, and electrical systems were expanded, and more than one hundred new buildings were constructed.[28] Despite these many changes, the barbed wire fence that had surrounded St. Luke's was not altered: it was left in place. There had also been internal barbed wire fences within the camp, but these were almost entirely removed.[29] This goes to show that even though the barbed wire fence that enclosed Israel's central reception camp was originally constructed by the British, it was willingly retained by the Jewish Agency. In the overhaul that took place when St. Luke's was transformed into Shaar Ha'aliya, it could have been removed along with the internal fences, but the Jewish Agency saw that it had a role to play: "One of the aims of the camp is the isolation of the new immigrant from the moment he arrives until after the medical examination, the results of which are received by the medical services. The isolation is the only guarantee to protect the Israeli Yishuv from epidemics and disease that could have flooded the country as a result of the mass immigration."[30] This argument made a lot of sense in its time. Historians' accounts of this period convey an atmosphere of panic, crisis, and despair among the people working in immigrant health.[31] They essentially tell a story of a wave of immigration that not only was unprecedentedly large and fast but also had extremely high rates of disease. Responsibility for this then fell on an utterly overwhelmed health care system that suffered from a shortage of funds and a shortage of hospital beds. The health care workers, the media, and eventually, the public became terrified that there would be outbreaks of serious epidemics. They saw people—including the children, the sick, the elderly—cramped together in immigrant camps in terrible conditions.[32] Even though the Jewish community in Palestine had previously taken in large waves of immigrants, this was unlike anything they had ever seen before, and the health care workers felt utterly unprepared for what they were facing. The arriving immigrants were exhausted and physically depleted. They needed attention and care. The lists of problems included malnutrition, tuberculosis, ringworm and trachoma, physical disabilities, frailty, and mental illnesses.[33] Throughout the country, there was a terrifying spike in infant mortality, which, reports show, was disproportionately high among the new immigrants.[34] Historian Avi Picard reached a clear conclusion: "The medical problems in the mass *aliyah* [immigration] were enormous. They were among the first factors to make Israelis uncomfortable with immigration."[35]

The evidence we have reinforces this picture of enormous medical problems and a serious concern about the spread of infectious disease. We know that a full 10 percent of all the immigrants from 1948 to 1951 needed to be hospitalized immediately. We also know that a huge number of the immigrants in the first years were Holocaust survivors (70 percent of the immigrants from 1948 to 1949) whose terrible experiences had left them physically and psychologically battered.[36] They suffered from high rates of malnutrition, chronic diseases (such as tuberculosis), and mental illness.[37] Various groups of the immigrants from Arab and Muslim countries were also very sick. For example, Avi Picard has written that sixteen thousand of the forty-six thousand immigrants from Yemen needed to be hospitalized as soon as they arrived in Israel.[38] Their arduous immigration experience and the cramped, unsanitary conditions in the transit camp in Aden had left the Yemenite community sick with intestinal and urinary parasites, malaria, trachoma, and tuberculosis.[39] Malaria and intestinal and urinary parasites were also prevalent among immigrants from Iraq, whereas immigrants from North Africa had high rates of trachoma, ringworm, and tuberculosis.[40] One illuminating perspective is that in certain villages in the Atlas Mountains, trachoma was so common "that it was not even considered an illness."[41]

Despite clear agreement between scholars on the severity of the health crisis, the evidence by and large gives dramatic and startling glimpses but not a complete picture. Historian Sachlav Stoler-Liss declared that "a mapping of the state of health during the mass immigration is not an easy task." She explains that the reason we only have patchy information is because we have to rely on the data published by the Central Bureau of Statistics, which, for those early years, is limited and poorly organized. There is no uniformity in their data, the categories and tables they provide are inconsistent and lacking.[42] To the extent that the data allowed it, Stoler-Liss set out to compile the most comprehensive list, to date, of the incidence of disease during the mass immigration. Her documentation, along with supplementary information, gives a clearer understanding of the epidemiology of the mass immigration. The contagious diseases that were tracked were dysentery and diphtheria, tuberculosis, polio, malaria, syphilis and gonorrhea, ringworm, and trachoma.[43]

The situation in Shaar Ha'aliya was similar to, though not exactly the same as, the larger picture found in the country. Trachoma, tuberculosis, syphilis, head lice, and scabies were some of the main diseases that were tracked. Malaria and polio, two of the three epidemics to hit Israel in these years, were not prevalent in Shaar Ha'aliya.[44] Stoler-Liss has concluded that there were indeed "several serious diseases where the rates of infection/illness among the immigrants were significantly higher"[45] than in the Yishuv. This was because of so many factors in their immigration experience, both before they left their home countries and after they arrived in Israel, that negatively impacted the health of Israel's immigrants: preexisting conditions from their countries of origin; the living conditions and quality of health care in their countries of origin; the difficult transit conditions encountered during migration; the crowded, unhygienic environments of Israel's temporary housing; and the nutritionally deficient diets of Israel's austerity period.[46]

A major concern was whether the Israeli medical system was equipped to care for so many very sick people, since, as soon as the immigrants arrived in Israel and became new citizens, they were immediately eligible for state-subsidized health care.[47] By 1948, the Israeli health care system was already well-established and—although certainly facing many grave challenges—was relatively well-functioning. On the day Ben-Gurion announced the establishment of the state, Israel had numerous public and private hospitals, four different sick funds, 2,500 doctors, and two thousand hospital beds.[48] They also had a larger network to rely on: soon after gaining independence, the State of Israel became linked to existing international health and aid organizations, signing an agreement with the United Nations Children's Fund (UNICEF) in 1948 and joining the World Health Organization (WHO) in 1949.[49] The WHO and UNICEF filled a vacuum in the field of public health that had been left by the departure of the British Mandate authorities. They played leading roles in public health policy during the mass immigration, offering "advice, aid, technical and substantive assistance, professional training and particularly help formulating active health policy." Their help was focused on the prevention and treatment of infectious diseases.[50]

Although the Israeli health care system had this help, as well as experience in caring for new immigrants from the Mandate period, it underwent a jarring shift from having absorbed 1,500 immigrants per month under the British to absorbing up to 10,000 per month during the mass immigration.[51] Avraham Sternberg served as director of Israel's Immigrant Health Services from 1949 to 1953. In his memoir, he describes a health care system that was materially, physically, and psychologically unprepared to treat so many patients: "The numbers alone, as fantastic as they were, are far from expressing the extent of the problems that came from the mass absorption [. . .] as the waves of immigration intensified we were sometimes faced with medical questions that up until then we had only learned about in books [. . .] The medical problems were many and varied."[52] The health care workers who were responsible for caring for the immigrants were depleted and completely overwhelmed: "Those of us in the Immigrant Health Services went on in our simple manner and we were no longer alarmed, since from the start we were alarmed to the very core of our being—to the point of despair."[53] The atmosphere of alarm is evident. Yet whether the epidemiological data actually supports a medical justification for a quarantine is certainly a question worth considering. The diseases found and tracked in Shaar Ha'aliya were not deemed "quarantinable" in Israel at the time.[54] As far as numbers go, most cases were head lice and trachoma. The former (which has to be distinguished from body lice / scabies and *was* distinguished from body lice in Shaar Ha'aliya, which was much less prevalent) is very contagious but not dangerous. As a leading cause of acquired blindness, particularly among children, trachoma was certainly both contagious and very dangerous.[55] This is also true of tuberculosis, which was also a serious concern in Shaar Ha'aliya. However, the treatment for these diseases, both in Shaar Ha'aliya and throughout Israel, followed international procedures and guidelines. Despite significant financial and organizational setbacks, the efforts were well-organized and efficient. With such organized treatment, was a quarantine actually necessary? It could be argued that the isolation was a preemptive measure, that only in hindsight can we see it was unnecessary, since, at the time, they could not know if there would be outbreaks of more ominous diseases such as smallpox or cholera. But I would argue that what we are seeing here is a different phenomenon: the environment of fear created an exaggerated sense of how threatening the people and their diseases really were as well as an exaggerated perspective on what the barrier was actually doing to isolate them.

A Sort of Quarantine Station

In November 1950, Yehuda Weisberger wrote to Kalman Levin (then director of the Absorption Department's Haifa office), describing how neither the fence nor the police guards were able to prevent people from entering and exiting the camp: "This guard does not prevent the new immigrants, with the help of their families outside, from damaging the fences and sneaking out through the ruptures."[56] In a later letter that deals with the same problem, Weisberger suggested that perhaps it was the Holocaust survivors who were predominantly responsible for this phenomenon: "There are among them [the immigrants], particularly those who come from European countries, who are skilled at burglarizing fences, who manage to leave the camp through the holes, despite the guards."[57] A former Shaar Ha'aliya employee recalled how the barbed wire and the police guards could not prevent the flow of unregulated movement in and out of the camp.[58] In one instance, a reporter from the newspaper *Davar* was stopped by the camp guards after breaking in through the fence.[59] In their 1950 report, an organization called "The Committee for the Study of Immigrants and Their Absorption" referred to both the quarantine and the breached fence in the same section without addressing the possibility that perhaps this meant that the quarantine was not particularly effective:

> The Shaar Ha'aliya camp is a sort of quarantine station. Leaving the camp is forbidden and a sharp, thick, barbed wire fence serves as a barrier between the camp residents and the world outside. But in fact, the new immigrants escape through holes and the camp authorities are abstaining from posting guards all along the fence so that it doesn't conjure associations of the closed camps infamously remembered from the days of the last war. The various "guests" that enter the camp, either with or without a permit, keep the 50 guards busy with their criminal activity and bring the prisons clients. Suspicious characters prey on innocent girls. The abundance of novelties dizzies them and weakens their self-control and their moral boundaries.[60]

This report encapsulates the many conflicts contained by this fence. The camp was enclosed by a forceful barrier, a "sharp, thick, barbed wire fence." The immigrants' isolation was intentional, leaving was "forbidden," and they were being separated from "the world outside." The negative implications of this space are clear, with the fear of "associations of the closed camps infamously remembered from the days of the last war." And there is that link to health, describing Shaar Ha'aliya as a quarantine but not entirely. Shaar Ha'aliya was a "sort of" quarantine station. On the one hand, it was closed, threatening, and isolating. And yet, apparently, it also wasn't because "the new immigrants escape through holes."

Overall, the camp administration estimated that 1 percent of the immigrants who went through Shaar Ha'aliya evaded the administrative process by slipping out through the fence.[61] But this number doesn't take into account people like Sylvia Meltzer and the many others who were accounted for and who didn't actually evade the administrative process but who just went back and forth through the fence. That number would be much higher. Moreover, some of the people were, perhaps, "escaping" as the previous report suggested, yet the term *escaping*—while not completely untrue—is misleading, since it suggests desperation, one-directional flight, and a threat of punishment. People weren't sneaking out of Shaar Ha'aliya at night to avoid being caught: photographs of people maneuvering through the fence were taken in daylight. Cutting through the wire did not need a complicated procedure with tools or middle-men: you just had to maneuver yourself under or through it. There's no indication that people were injured from the spikes, and there's no indication that people would have been afraid or even hesitant to break through the fence because they were concerned about being caught. Once when a police guard stopped a family as they tried to go through the fence, he rode up to them on his bicycle—no gun, handcuffs, or arrests—and directed them to return to the camp.[62] Very possibly they just went back through at another time when the guard was not looking. The fence was an unpleasant obstacle, but getting out of the camp through its holes was neither a stealthy nor a life-threatening endeavor.

The people who were going in and out through the Shaar Ha'aliya fence were largely going on with their lives, and they just didn't let the fence get in their way. They visited family, went to the city for entertainment, looked for jobs, and bought products on the black market. In many cases, they came back to the camp later in the day. In other cases, they were breaking *in* to Shaar Ha'aliya just because it was easier than going through the main entrance. Some of the people breaking in were those "criminal guests" described by the "Committee for the Study of Immigrants." But it is hard to say just how truly "criminal" these people were, since some of the people who the police labeled this way were other immigrants (particularly from Iraq) who came from outside of the camp to help organize protests.[63] There was crime in the camp, but whether this came from people on the outside, sneaking in, is unsubstantiated. There were also people like Sylvia

Meltzer, who simply and matter-of-factly broke in and out regularly. It is likely that there were people who were upset at what they found at Shaar Ha'aliya and, deciding to leave, went out though holes in the fence. But even in these cases, the term *escaping* falls short, since there were no repercussions to leaving. People were not shot at, put in prison, or deported. The only obstacle put in their way was the fence itself and then later, also a small group of police guards with little power. The "sharp, thick, barbed wire fence" that was an intentional part of Shaar Ha'aliya's structure and that was meant to act as a deterrent, to a large extent, failed. So many of the people it was meant to contain simply ignored it.

IMMIGRANT PROTEST

Controlling the fence was not the only way that immigrants asserted their power. Immigrants throughout Israel were making their displeasure known through noncompliance and rebellion.[64] This spirit of protest was very much alive in Shaar Ha'aliya. The new immigrants at the camp protested through letters to the press, letters of complaint to the camp administration, physical and verbal acts of rebellion, use of physical aggression, and organized demonstrations. There were those who staged large rallies, such as the group of around one hundred Iraqi immigrants who protested the discrimination they encountered and the preferential treatment of Europeans.[65] There were those who, upset about the housing placements they were given, refused to leave the camp when they were told.[66] Others became violent, physically attacking the clerks who were responsible for their processing.[67] Countless others wrote letters of complaint about camp life and policy. In language that was often biting, they got the immigrants' voices heard by the camp administration, by the press, by the public. A new immigrant wrote to the *Jerusalem Post* that life in Shaar Ha'aliya made him and his peers feel "as if they were prisoners, and not immigrants."[68] One man complained about the clerks at Shaar Ha'aliya: "It is about time . . . that the people who are responsible for the immigrants at Shaar Ha'aliya learn to treat them like living human beings."[69] Yet another immigrant brought attention to the shabby surroundings: "Shaar Aliya is an awfully filthy place . . . the administration is very much responsible for allowing such conditions to continue."[70]

In this pervasive spirit of protest, the immigrants also challenged the health care system at Shaar Ha'aliya and, in several instances, successfully brought about change. One notable case was a hunger strike by tuberculosis (TB) patients. Two huts on the camp premises were set aside for immigrants with TB while they waited to be transferred to hospitals.[71] Like the rest of the camp, these two huts were spartan and uncomfortable: "The crowding was great. The sanitation was disgraceful. In the summer it was very hot. In the winter it was very cold."[72] But an alternative location was hard to find. TB was a grave concern during the mass immigration. It was one of three major epidemics to hit Israel in its formative years, along with malaria and polio.[73] The rate of infection was high, the rate of death from the disease was high, and for the first years of the mass immigration, there was a consistent and dire shortage of beds for the hospitalization of TB patients. As a result, TB patients could not be transferred anywhere better, and their stay in Shaar Ha'aliya dragged on. Then in 1950, one of Shaar Ha'aliya's two busiest years, a group of immigrants with tuberculosis refused to accept this standstill; and they went on a hunger strike to protest their living conditions. This group of around eighty people was made up of mostly young adults from Europe, with a few immigrants from North Africa. One witness describes the protesters, their "pale faces," as they "sat sad and despairing."[74] By refusing to eat, the patients wanted to force the officials to relocate them out of Shaar Ha'aliya into a hospital where they hoped they would receive better treatment and better conditions. The strike lasted for two days. Through this act of protest, the immigrants gained the attention, sympathy, and respect of leading health and immigration officials. And although the resources at the time were extremely limited, two weeks later they were transferred out of Shaar

Ha'aliya to a makeshift TB hospital in the town of Pardesiya. Not only were these people very sick, they were also newly arrived immigrants, but that did not stop them from being empowered to organize as a group and successfully fight and change the conditions they encountered.

There were others who did not organize as a group like the hunger strikers but acted individually to defy Shaar Ha'aliya's various rules, as happened when one woman "stole" her ailing son away from the children's health care facility:

> We arrived at Shaar Ha'aliya. It was very, very hard. Very hard. My son immediately got dysentery. With blood. He was two years old. Two years old. They took him to this kind of hospital. There was a hospital. All the children were sick. In Shaar Ha'aliya. And they took a sort of . . . house, and there they put all the [sick] children. Every day two or three died. Every day, every day. And they gave them this sort of food, and we were in these tents, we were there in Shaar Ha'aliya. And I saw that they weren't letting people into the hospital, to see the child, and I saw . . . his whole bottom was red . . . they didn't see it . . . there were so many children. So I went . . . me and my husband . . . we put a ladder and we went in through the window and I took the child. I took the child . . . to the tent.

Once she and her husband had their son back with them in their own tent, they cared for him by themselves, nursing him back to health:

> And every day . . . rice. I gave him rice and here, I took care of everything . . . his bottom . . . and I gave him everything that you need to eat when he is sick like that. And later a doctor came to where I was in the tent. And he said, [. . .] with what right did you take the child? He is very sick. I said: They don't see, he's crying. I saw through the window he was crying. So many children and only two nurses, I said. [The doctor said] sign that you have taken your son. So I signed. I signed and I

took the child. Day and night I didn't sleep. I gave him this and that and
water and tea. They don't give all this! He was dehydrated. So, some time
went by and I see that the child is better. That he is getting well here.[75]

This woman described how potential conflict, stemming from this act of
defiance, was resolved after a doctor confronted her about the removal
of her son. Having a language in common with the doctor was a crucial
part of how this scenario played out: after speaking to him in Yiddish with
the help of an ad hoc interpreter, she managed to persuade the doctor to
let the child stay with her.[76] She kept her son with her, taking care of him
herself, and under her care, he eventually got well. It is a fantastic account
that, it would seem, was not unique to this one incident. In a 1950 report
on Shaar Ha'aliya, similar scenarios are described, with parents crowded
around the windows of the children's hospital, refusing to leave their children alone and, in several cases, breaking in and forcibly removing their
children from the hospital premises.

> People crowded around the windows of the hospital. It was explained
> to us that these are the parents of the sick children who don't budge
> from the place and watch over their children day and night because they
> distrust the hospital's treatment methods. In their eyes the therapeutic
> diet is considered to be a starvation diet that threatens the lives of their
> children. There were incidents where parents broke into the hospital
> and forcibly removed their children from the hands of the caregivers.
> It's possible that sub-conscious memories from the Holocaust bring out
> the parents' fears and unsettle their trust. It's also possible that this is
> caused by differences in culture and lifestyle from the peoples different
> countries of origin, because modern medical methods are up against a
> wall of preconceptions.[77]

The immigrants who came to Israel in the 1950s are often depicted as
victims,[78] and certainly these are stories about hardship and discrimination. But they are also stories about boldness and empowerment. Whether

writing letters, refusing to leave the camp when told, staging a hunger strike, or climbing through windows to reclaim one's child, the immigrants at Shaar Ha'aliya were significantly empowered, forcing change and refusing the conditions that were imposed upon them. Each of these cases of defiance suggests that the immigrants believed that their arrival in the new state came with certain entitlements: entitlement to particular standards of health care and standards of living, entitlement to parental autonomy, and—as seen by the breached fence—entitlement to freedom of movement.[79]

In much the same way that the TB patients protested against their conditions of health care and a mother refused to have her sick son taken away from her, the immigrants at Shaar Ha'aliya fought against being contained inside the barbed wire fence. But this protest was longer, more drawn out and gradual.[80] The immigrants did not stage one large rebellion over this. Camp residents didn't come together at a certain time to pull the fence down. Instead, daily, over time, and with relative ease, they simply defied it. One man lifted the wire for his friend to crawl under. Another elderly couple grasped one another as they stepped over the wire that was pushed down. The young girl Sylvia, when visiting her family, only ever entered and exited the camp through a hole in the fence; and she did so as an unhesitant matter-of-fact action. Gradually and without fanfare, the Shaar Ha'aliya immigrants created a situation that prompted one official to say, "In theory the camp is closed, but in reality it is open to all."[81] Breaking through the fence must be seen as an empowered act of protest because, in this way, the immigrants actively created an alternative to the situation they were given. It wasn't confusion or resignation that led them to go in and out of the barbed wire barrier. Even when done calmly or matter-of-factly, this was a conscious, physical way to expand the boundaries placed around them.

HELP GUARD THE QUARANTINE

The defiance of the fence frustrated the police who, as a result, had to work even harder to control what was going on in the camp. This issue highlights how trying their work was. Like all Shaar Ha'aliya employees, the police were under incredible pressure in this epicenter of the mass immigration, where they were part of an underprepared, overwhelmed system. The ineffective fence only made things harder for them. In the first months that Shaar Ha'aliya was open, it was, in fact, run with no police surveillance. In July 1949, Giora Josephtal (then head of the Jewish Agency's Absorption Department) criticized this absence and the internal squabbles that were causing the delay. He insisted that police be immediately positioned, declaring, "Shaar Ha'aliya needs police more than any other immigration centre."[82] When a police station was finally opened in July 1949, it consisted of fifty-nine guards whose job was to do the following:

1. Maintain order and oversee security
2. Guard the quarantine[83]

The relations between the camp administration and the Shaar Ha'aliya police unit appear to have been initially positive,[84] but by January 1951, Yehuda Weisberger sent a report to the Absorption Department's northern office that was fiercely critical of the Shaar Ha'aliya guards. He belittled the guards' character, referring to them as "poor human material." He described them as immigrants who came to their jobs in Shaar Ha'aliya only after they had been rejected from all other employment frameworks. He accused them of drunkenness, theft, and lewd behavior. Finally, he declared them to be causing the camp "moral damage." In his view, the police's behavior was so damaging that, had it been possible, he would have run the camp without them. While Weisberger made a point of saying that not every guard was of such "poor human material," he insisted that the good ones were few in number and of little influence. And he wrote that as far as the quarantine was concerned, the camp police had "failed a bitter failure."[85]

One month later, Shefi, the overseeing officer for the Shaar Ha'aliya police station, composed a similarly rancorous response. While he opened by admitting to serious disciplinary problems within the police, he deflected the blame onto Weisberger and the Jewish Agency: "If there is some degree of the neglect described by Mr. Weisberger, and if anyone is to be blamed for it, there is no doubt that it must be the camp director himself and the general manager of the Jewish Agency's absorption camps, who haven't lifted a finger to construct the camp as planned in 1949, so that it could be used for the purpose that it was intended, despite constantly repeated promises that have not been fulfilled even to the smallest extent."[86] Shefi blamed the Jewish Agency for not having made any technical adjustments to the camp infrastructure to accommodate the growing population, resulting in a scenario where eight thousand people were living in a space equipped for four to five thousand. He insisted that, no matter how hard the guards may have tried, they could absolutely never get the quarantine under control as long as the fence was so shabby and ineffective: "In spite of all the widespread disciplinary and instructional efforts, it is not in the guards' power to conduct proper surveillance around the fence—despite their good intentions and preparation."[87] He blamed the Jewish Agency for not keeping its promises to build a proper fence, for changing the concept of the camp without making necessary adaptations to the physical space, and for not heeding his recommendations for camp structure and location. He also blamed Weisberger for using the police guards as scapegoats for what were actually the blunderings of the Jewish Agency.

As far as the system by which the officers were employed, with no job security and dismissals monthly, he writes, "You will agree with me that in these conditions it is impossible to maintain order and discipline." On the issue Weisberger referred to as "poor human material," Shefi does not argue. His explanation for this is that many of the people working on the Shaar Ha'aliya police force had been in Israel for less than a year and were stationed at Shaar Ha'aliya after only a few months of experience in the police force.[88] Shefi does not dwell on the shortcomings of the police officers; rather, he says, "But these are the Jews we have, and we have no others." Ultimately, he describes an internal system so fundamentally dysfunctional that it would have been impossible for the police to have had any significant impact.

Following his report, Shefi's superior, Y. Nahmias, appears to have taken the complaints seriously by sending Giora Josephtal a letter Shefi had written that documented the troubles with the fence, the subsequent inability of the police to do effective work, and the Jewish Agency's accountability for not having already solved this problem. Shefi writes, "The police is forced into an ongoing struggle with the thousands of immigrants inside the camp and the hundreds of people outside the camp who are trying to get past the fence for mutual meetings and visits . . . This situation makes it so that the police force does not have even a minimal possibility of containing the crowd and establishing order in the camp."[89] As in the letter to Weisberger, Shefi emphasizes again and again the need for the Jewish Agency to build an effective fence. He ends by threatening that, should the fence not be fixed within a month, he would "remove the police from the area and release himself of all the responsibility for the camp security."[90]

Shefi had actually written this report in August 1950, at which point he insisted that, without a proper, sturdy fence, they could not be responsible for guarding the camp.[91] This request was rejected by Josephtal, out of concern for how the public would react: "The first suggestion [to build a wall around the camp] is unacceptable to us as, I imagine, it also is for you. The impression that we are receiving immigrants in the courtyard of a 'prison,' would raise up the entire public and its institutions against us."[92] Following Josephtal's forthright rejection of the wall proposal in 1950, the problem did not disappear. The fact that the 1950 letter was re-sent in 1951 and the correspondence that followed seem to suggest that Weisberger's

1951 report gave the police incentive to push for action—in addition to, perhaps, a desire to have their situation understood in the higher echelons of power.

In 1951, after the report was sent a second time, Nahmias let Shefi know that his response to Weisberger was being taken seriously. He expressed his sympathy with the situation Shefi was in and agreed that "in the existing conditions there could be no way to bring order to the camp in an accept-able manner."[93] The 1951 letters seem to have finally had the result that the 1950 letters did not. Police files show that by April 1951, a wall was being built: "Pressure that the Shore and Border Police's commanding officer put on the Jewish Agency has proved fruitful, and they have started building a brick wall around the camp that will make the guards' job easier and will help guard the quarantine."[94] Through this exchange, we see how the act of going in and out through a hole in the fence, which Sylvia Meltzer had described with such ease, was a serious point of contention for the people whose job it was to stop that from happening. Yehuda Weisberger saw this as yet another lapse on a long list of faults for the police, which—in his mind—was a struggling, lame body. For Shefi, it was a sign of the impossible situation that he and his staff were being put in because his Jewish Agency superiors were afraid of "what it would look like" to fortify the fence. Shefi wanted them to acknowledge how difficult the police work was, and he wanted them to recognize that the police would not be able to succeed on their own, that certain circumstances set them up to fail, and that certain measures would have to be taken for their work to have any efficacy, which led him to ask that the fence be reinforced. Equally telling, however, are the things the police did *not* ask for. They did not ask for the power to fine people breaking through the fence. They did not want to arrest them; and they did not request permission to physically intimidate them, beat them, or shoot them. Through this push and pull, these vari-ous agents of the new state were negotiating how far Israeli state authority was willing to go to enforce the physical barrier of the quarantine. A police presence was accepted, but it was limited. A barbed wire fence and then a wall were ultimately accepted, but they were not without controversy. In the larger context of nation building, the fence allowed people to wrestle with the many layers and dimensions of Israel's boundaries.

The story of Shaar Ha'aliya's quarantine began with the physical structure of the fence. It was part of an environment of widespread fear of disease and, as such, had a role to play in "the isolation of the immigrant from the moment he arrives."[95] But a defining part of this structure was its permeability and the struggle over its control. The immigrants who went under and over it easily and constantly were asserting their considerable power by refusing to be isolated from the rest of Israel. But for the police, this permeability was a major concern. Their job was to keep order in a place of disarray and to guard the quarantine, and as long as people were breaking in and out of the fence, this was nearly impossible. As we will see, this struggle over space was only part of the problem. At this time, the very idea of a barbed wire fence for Jews, in Israel, was a source of intense conflict.

CHAPTER 3

Meaning

In April 1951, Shabtai Keshev, a reporter who wrote under the name K. Shabtai, sat down to compose an article on Shaar Ha'aliya. Keshev was a Holocaust survivor who had been imprisoned in the Kovno ghetto for four years, and he made his feelings clear: this place and its barbed wire fence were a shameful sight. "Shaar Ha'aliya has become the first stain on the country's name, the first to poison the new immigrant's soul. . . . Barbed wire fences surround the camp, fences that are a penetrated wall on the one hand and a prison on the other."[1] Around the same time that this article came out, Shefi (Shaar Ha'aliya's overseeing police officer) was drafting his own reports about the camp guards, which had a very different take on the Shaar Ha'aliya fence. What Keshev described as a "prison," Shefi presented simply as a logical safeguard. Unsurprisingly, from his perspective as the man responsible for keeping order and guarding the quarantine, the barbed wire fence was a straightforward matter that he did not question. It was a natural and welcome measure of policy and order.[2]

Shabtai and Shefi were not alone. Many people, whether Jewish Agency officials, camp employees, international and local journalists, or members of the public, all had something to say about the quarantine. This chapter explores what they were saying.[3] These texts make it clear that, just as there was a physical push and pull surrounding the fence, there was also one that was conceptual and verbal; whether within themselves or between one another, people struggled with and could not agree upon any one interpretation or meaning of the Shaar Ha'aliya quarantine. Some were like Shefi. For them, the Shaar Ha'aliya fence was a comfort, a measure that suggested security, keeping the grave dangers of disease and immigration at bay. This meaning of quarantine is protective. It ties in directly to what Alan M. Kraut has called the "double helix" of immigration and disease, two themes that are linked and deeply feared in the societies that receive newcomers. For many people in the Yishuv, the immigrants and their diseases were perceived as threats and quarantine and biomedicine were perceived as shields. Others were like Shabtai. For them, the fence was a shameful and embarrassing symbol of isolation that threatened the social fabric of the new society. This meaning of quarantine is punitive. It holds on to the idea that the Jewish state was supposed to be a symbol of inclusion for all Jews, whereas a camp enclosed by a barbed wire fence symbolized exclusion and persecution.

These positions are not always dichotomous; people bounced opinions around and moderated them in some cases only to intensify them elsewhere—sometimes even in the same text. Nevertheless, several important ideas come through: (1) The "setting apart" of new immigrants in a camp behind barbed wire hit a nerve in Israeli society even before Shaar Ha'aliya was opened because of associations with the camps of the Holocaust. But it was also, just as quickly, accepted and defended through the logic of disease and quarantine. (2) The fact that the same people who were defending the quarantine as medically necessary also knew that it wasn't successfully keeping people out ties into Wendy Brown's theoretical work on walls as theatrical displays of power meant to obfuscate vulnerability. The meaning of the fence, and the discussion surrounding its meaning, comes down to fear, fences, and medicine: the context was one of fear of contagion, the fence was a sign of control in the face of that fear, and medicine (the defending logic behind a quarantine) was a reassuring and powerful authority. (3) Finally, one of the most important meanings ascribed to quarantine in this discourse is as an alternative to the camps of Europe: displaced peoples (DP) or concentration camps. When people, inevitably and repeatedly, commented on similarities between Shaar Ha'aliya's appearance and concentration camps of the Holocaust, "quarantine" was offered as an alternative conceptual frame, as a way to say, "You see a fence and an isolation that harm, but you should see a fence and an isolation that heal."

This chapter disentangles the threads of the Shaar Ha'aliya / quarantine discourse while shining a light on the entanglements that still persist; there are blurred boundaries and blatant contradictions throughout. The story that emerges reinforces Shaar Ha'aliya's place within a broader frame of quarantine, where we find both an overlap between modern systems of coerced isolation (a prison / a quarantine / a processing camp) as well as fuzzy borders between physical and social "contagion." Moreover, what also emerges is a sense of the depth of this conflict, as people struggled with what it meant for the Jewish state to have a fenced-in quarantine for these particular people at this particular time and place.

From outside Israel, Looking at Shaar Ha'aliya

In August 1949, the *New York Herald Tribune* published a series of five articles that followed the journey of hundreds of immigrants on the ship the *Atzmaut* (Hebrew for "independence") as it traveled from Bari, Italy, to Haifa. Ruth Gruber, the author of these articles, was a renowned writer and photojournalist from New York who had begun writing for the *New York Herald Tribune* while living in Germany in the 1930s. Her life's work was devoted to critical political and social issues of her time: the rise of Hitler and Europe's growing expressions of anti-Semitism in the 1930s, the Nuremberg trials, the settlement of veterans returning to the United States, and the plight of Holocaust survivors and Jewish refugees around the world. Gruber's reporting of the story of the *Exodus* in 1947—a ship of Jewish DP's from Germany that was turned away from British-controlled Palestine—was responsible for the international attention the story

received. Similarly, in 1944, Gruber's involvement was critical in arrang-
ing for one thousand Jewish refugees to get temporary admission—and
later citizenship—in the United States. Therefore when Gruber set out
for Haifa on the *Atzmaut*, she was already a proven global advocate for
the refugees she was accompanying.[4]

The 1949 series on the *Atzmaut* is humanizing and dramatic. The
articles' emphatic titles lay out a story of refugees rejected by Europe and
North Africa arriving in their rightful and welcoming home of Israel. It
begins with "Sailing for the Promised Land" and ends, four days later, with
"Refugees' Landing in Israel: 'It's Our Land, It Belongs to Us.'"[5] Gruber
focused on the immigrants' stories as they were told to her on the trip over
and their hopes and fears about starting a new life. The series ends with
a final article describing the first few hours after the emotional arrival in
Israel: "They crowded the deck for hours to catch their first glimpse of the
Holy Land. At 2 o'clock, jammed against the gunwales they stood, singing
'Hatikvah.' It was the song the Jews had sung in the ghettos and on the
death march to the gas chambers. It was the song the Jews sang when they
ran the British blockade. Now it is the anthem of the new state, and Israel's
newest immigrants sang it with choked voices." One woman's story highlighted how, after going through hell, arriving in Israel was an extraordinary feeling of finally belonging somewhere:

> A woman who had lost her entire family in the crematoria said to me,
> "I can't believe it yet; we're really home. No more running. It's our
> own land. Nobody can say to me anymore, 'Jews not wanted here.' This
> belongs to me. I don't know how to say this to you, but for the first time
> since 1939, my heart feels light. Do you know what it means not to run
> any more, not to be hounded by brutes? To be able to breathe again? To
> know you're wanted? That's how I feel now. Like a person who's wanted
> and welcome. Like a human being."

Gruber described Shaar Ha'aliya as "an elongated jumble of tents and
wooden barracks along the Mediterranean." Then in the last paragraph

of the article, which ends her entire series, she wrote, "Sha'ar Aliyah, where the people stay from four to ten days, is to be turned into a quarantine camp so that any infectious diseases can be isolated. The immigrants received a thorough medical examination and in a week or two were to be transferred to one of three places: a permanent immigration camp, a farm colony, or a former Arab village. The few with relatives or friends with apartments had no housing problems." Gruber makes no direct allusion to the barbed wire fence. Her reference to quarantine is fleeting and accepting. It implies that it is normative and inconsequential, and perhaps—after going through the Holocaust—for these people, a quarantine camp really was the least of their worries.

For Raymond Cartier, however, the symbol of barbed wire was not inconsequential. Cartier, a French journalist and author, came to Israel in 1949 to cover Israel's early development. The result was a long article published in the August 1949 issue of the popular French magazine *Paris-Match*.[6] At this time, Cartier was already a well-known columnist. But it was only seven years later, in 1956, that he became famous for his arguments against maintaining French colonies. Cartier's main argument against the colonies was that they were an economic burden and that, rather than pay for them, France would do better investing the money in the metropole. This anticolonial position, which would come to be known as "Cartierism," was first articulated in a series of essays Cartier published for *Paris-Match* in 1956.[7] Although his earlier piece about Israel deals with a different space and subject, it is possible to see the pragmatic and critical worldviews that Cartier would become synonymous with coming through in his gaze on the new Jewish state.

Cartier, like Gruber, wrote about the immigrant encounter with Israel. His long and compelling article combines several pages of text with large photographs. He remarked upon developments in Israeli industry and scholarship and the general challenges that the new immigrants faced: the housing shortage, a lack of private living space, cultural gaps, and the obstacles to integration. While Gruber's articles depict immigrants who were largely reconciled with the difficulties they expected to encounter in Israel ("Immigrants on the Atzmaut Are Prepared to Face Austerity and Hardships for Life of Hope"), Cartier, on the other hand, depicts less reconciliation. He brought attention to an important theme: the clash between the ideal of immigrating to the Jewish state and the very difficult reality.

Accordingly, Cartier emphasized that Shaar Ha'aliya was a problem. He wrote that the new immigrants arrived full of hope for what awaited them in Israel only to find what they had thought that they had left behind them: camps surrounded by barbed wire. Already in the fall of 1949, only a few months after Shaar Ha'aliya had opened, Shaar Ha'aliya is being associated with Holocaust imagery. But Cartier makes an important distinction between the camps of Europe and Israel: "These are camps of hope instead of camps of death, but they are still 'camps.'" This is not Gruber's simple acceptance of the isolation. Cartier makes no reference to health and quarantine as justifications. Not only does he see the barbed wire as punitive; he associates it with the worst kind of imprisonment. But he moderated himself by saying that this camp offered possibility and life and not the horrors of the Holocaust.

Robert Capa's view of Shaar Ha'aliya's fence was closer to Cartier's critique than it was to Gruber's acceptance. A Hungarian-born Jew who had begun working as a photographer in Berlin in the 1930s, by the time Capa photographed Shaar Ha'aliya he was already one of the world's most celebrated photojournalists, especially known for his images of war.[8] Capa first arrived in Israel in May 1948, after he was commissioned by *Life* magazine to document the establishment of the state. He left Israel in June 1948 but returned a few months later, in January 1949, to cover the country's postwar developments with his friend, the American journalist Irwin Shaw.[9] Capa's images from this time range greatly: there are portraits of politicians, families dancing happily in their Tel Aviv living rooms, Jewish agricultural workers eating in a Kibbutz dining hall riddled with bullet holes, and immigrants arriving at Shaar Ha'aliya.[10]

By all accounts, Robert Capa was moved by the refugees he saw arriving in Israel.[11] He also identified with them: he too was uprooted ("essentially a stateless person and perpetual refugee by temperament and profession"), and he too was a Jew.[12] But beyond these connections, which may have colored his encounter, it is clear from his images of people from across the world that Capa was fundamentally moved by the human condition and touched by human vulnerability.[13] A recurring theme in Capa's broad body of work, the plight of refugees clearly came in to play in his encounter at Shaar Ha'aliya. One of Capa's biographers, Alex Kershaw, describes Capa's photographs there of children, orphaned by the Holocaust, as "the most harrowing" of all thousands of "pictures he took of displaced children in his career."[14] For Capa, the barbed wire fence was a difficult image to accept in this setting. In an article to accompany his photographs, he wrote, "So the 'people of the barbed wire,' who have passed through scores of concentration and refugee camps in the last decade, reach the land of their dreams, only to be back once more behind barbed wire!"[15] The meaning here is clear: Shaar Ha'aliya's fence was a symbol of oppression. It evoked images of the Holocaust and DP camps and it dampened the hopeful arrival in the "Promised Land." No doubt Richard Whelan was correct in writing that "Capa was dismayed by the plight of these reluctant internees."[16]

Despite this unsettling imagery, Capa—like Cartier—goes on to describe a camp, and indeed a country, bustling with energy. People are moving out of Shaar Ha'aliya to start a new stage of life. He describes a country facing grave problems but filled with romantic possibility. Capa was buoyed by the immigrants themselves and "fascinated" by the way they were being integrated "into the life of the new nation."[17] He was amused by stories of people breaking out of the barbed wire to visit prostitutes.[18] He remarked on how the immigrants quickly settled into the camp routine.[19] And while his pictures show the hardships of refugee life, the difficulty of arriving in Shaar Ha'aliya, and the severity of its barbed wire enclosure, they also show people enjoying themselves, caring for one another, carrying on with

their lives, and interacting with simple normalcy.[20] Moreover, the photograph of the man crawling out under the barbed wire fence is not a simple
image of oppression. Through the lens of his camera, Robert Capa gave
the image more meaning. He pushes Raymond Cartier's idea (that this is
a camp of life) even further and—perhaps—adds a wink: this is a camp
of *chutzpah*. The fence may be a *symbol* of oppression, but the people are
not being oppressed.

Ruth Gruber, Raymond Cartier, and Robert Capa were all journalists
who had traveled across the globe documenting the human experience in
vastly different places during tumultuous times. They were all trained to
have a critical eye, and for a brief while in August 1949, they turned those
critical eyes on Israel's immigrants arriving at Shaar Ha'aliya.[21] With their
international outsiders' perspectives, they looked on with curiosity at this
phenomenon.[22] The fact that this story was being written about in great
detail in the *New York Herald Tribune*, *Paris-Match*, and *Illustrated* shows
that clearly it was of interest to the large audiences of widely read, international magazines. Each of these celebrated journalists mentioned the
quarantine and fence in some way and interpreted it differently. For Ruth
Gruber, the barbed wire fence seems not to have even made an impression.
She focused on the incredible hope that Israel gave the immigrants and
the "quarantine camp" of "elongated jumble of wooden barracks" in no
way dampened that hope. But for Cartier and Capa, it was more troubling.
They did not find resolution in the idea of "quarantine" and protection
from infectious diseases. They found resolution, hope, and even romance
in the larger context of the country and its peoples, but they were unsettled about what Shaar Ha'aliya's barbed wire structure conveyed, and they
were not the only ones.

FROM INSIDE ISRAEL, LOOKING AT SHAAR HA'ALIYA

The following year, in 1950, Yaakov Meridor, a member of Israel's right
wing party, Herut, stood up in the Knesset, the Israeli parliament, and

made a provocative statement: "Does the honourable minister know that, in appearance, the immigrant camp 'Shaar Ha'aliya' in Haifa gives the impression of a British concentration camp, or another concentration camp? Does not the honourable minister feel that it is not in accordance with the honour of the Jewish State to be holding new immigrants behind barbed wire?"[23] Like Cartier before him, Meridor draws attention to the similarities between the image of Shaar Ha'aliya and the European camps used for Jewish oppression and persecution. At the time of Meridor's comment, it had only been five years since World War II had ended, and Holocaust survivors made up a significant number of the immigrants to Israel. In this context, the image of Jews held in a camp was terrible, familiar, and immensely powerful.

It was not only members of the opposition party, Herut, who were making this association with the Holocaust as a way to challenge government policy. Even before Shaar Ha'aliya was opened, people were aware that it would be controversial. As part of discussions held by the Labor Zionist Mapai leadership in 1948, Giora Josephtal addressed these concerns: "Whether we like it or not, our processing camps will, to some extent, resemble the internment camps in Cyprus, and maybe even the internment camps in Germany."[24] For his part, Josephtal insisted that the fence was unavoidable: "There is no way to process and examine the immigrants if they are not initially concentrated in closed camps."[25] Here we see the beginning of what will become the Jewish Agency's recurrent justification for the fence: it is unfortunate but necessary. In this response, Josephtal does not mention disease. He appeals to a need for order. While he mentions the need to examine the immigrants in closed camps, he doesn't say that it is a medical necessity.

Three years later, we find echoes of the same justification intensified through the threat of disease. In March 1951, Kalman Levin wrote a letter to a Dr. Berman, who worked as director of a Tel Aviv high school. Dr. Berman had heard his students talk about how difficult an experience Shaar Ha'aliya had been for them, and he wrote Levin, it would seem, for the purpose of making his disapproval known. Levin responded, offering his own explanations for the points Berman had criticized. On the issue of the enclosure, he made an unequivocal statement: "The Shaar Ha'aliya camp has to be fenced and closed, as it is a quarantine. The Ministry of Health, Defence, Customs, Immigration and our department all demand that it be so. Were Dr. Berman to know of the number of diseases that we are treating at Shaar Ha'aliya among the immigrants, and among them the number of contagious diseases, you would also think differently and you would say, along with us, that our government must close the camp in a thorough manner for the sake of the Yishuv and for the sake of the immigrants."[26] In response to criticism of the fence, Levin acknowledged both the negative and the reassuring meanings of the image: "Perhaps from an emotional standpoint you are right. Because we are all opposed to the barbed wire fence [sic], which reminds us all of so much, but is there any alternative?"[27] Levin's explanation includes ideas that were central to the Jewish Agency's meaning of the quarantine—namely, that it was normative and essential: "One of the aims of the camp is the isolation of the new immigrant from the moment he arrives until after the medical examination, the results of which are received by the medical services. The isolation is the only guarantee to protect the Israeli Yishuv from epidemics and disease that could have flooded the country as a result of the great wave of immigration."[28] It is then no surprise that Yehuda Weisberger also explained it in a similar way. In 1950, a letter was published in the newspaper the *Jerusalem Post* that was extremely critical of Shaar Ha'aliya. The author was an immigrant from Bulgaria who went through the camp as part of his immigration process. After having been there for only a few days he was so appalled that he was moved to write a scathing and public account. He held nothing back. He said that Shaar Ha'aliya was an embarrassment to Israel, that arriving there made the immigrants lose their love for the land of their forefathers, and that instead of being welcomed as brethren, the immigrants were made to feel rejected and unwanted. The letter pinpointed specific problems in how the camp was run and made suggestions for changes that could be made to improve the living conditions. But the most dramatic assertion came right at the opening of the letter: "Next to the German concentration camps that I have heard about and read about, Shaar Ha'aliya is the worst place I have ever seen in my life." Here, again, Shaar Ha'aliya conjured images of the camps of the Holocaust. This letter does not make direct reference to the quarantine or the barbed wire, though by making an association with a concentration camp, the idea of oppression and forced containment is very bluntly present.[29]

The Jewish Agency asked Weisberger to reply. His response followed the pattern of many of his official letters; it was a long, point-by-point rebuttal of the issues raised in the complaint. He noted that when the immigrants arrived at the camp they actually received a warm greeting from the officials as well as an explanation of camp policy "in a language the immigrant understands." He defended the Shaar Ha'aliya staff and said that they were in a difficult position because the immigrants had unrealistic demands. The tone of this letter is often dismissive, patronizing, and then, finally, denigrating. Weisberger said that the author was "excessively emotional." He wrote that there were points that he simply wouldn't even bother answering, and he ignored the fact that many of the complaints were in fact absolutely accurate. He ended by suggesting that the man was mentally ill and that the problems described were true only in "the complainant's sick imagination."[30]

This letter prominently features the trope of "quarantine as a necessary measure of protection from disease." The following was Weisberger's response to the comment that Shaar Ha'aliya looked like a concentration camp: "There is no point in explaining to him [the author] the necessity for the existence of the quarantine that has been implemented to protect the health of the Yishuv from contagious diseases from overseas." Weisberger explained that they had tried to educate the public on the difference between Shaar Ha'aliya and camps outside of Israel; they used presentations, public relations, and publications to "blur" the associations that arose. And he used the same sort of reasoning that Josephtal and

Levin had used: the associations are unfortunate, but for the good of the public health, Shaar Ha'aliya has to be a fenced-in quarantine: "However, the basic fact remains the same. For a period of 5–6 days the immigrant stays closed inside a camp that is surrounded by a fence. There are a few people, especially those who, in the past, had been imprisoned in camps, for whom this brings up associations [with concentration camps]. As it is known, the immigrant leaves the camp as soon as the doctor determines that he is allowed to leave. And even if the immigrant does not grasp the necessity for the quarantine that does not mean that we should do away with it."[31] From the podium of the Knesset to the pages of national and international newspapers, immigrants, politicians, and journalists were saying—no less—that Israel's "gate of immigration" looked like a concentration camp. Ruth Gruber did not make this association. She mentioned quarantine in passing, as a normative, untroubling part of the immigration process. However, Josephtal, Levin, and Weisberger were well aware of how disturbing the image of the fence was, and they publically acknowledged that it was not ideal, but then they raised the issue of health. The immigrants were bringing diseases. These diseases threatened the Yishuv. The barbed wire fence controlled the spread of these diseases. Therefore the barbed wire fence was unfortunate but necessary.

Fear, Fences, and Medicine

What complicates this position, that the Shaar Ha'aliya quarantine was a necessary public health measure, is—of course—the man in Capa's photograph who is crawling under the barbed wire fence. At the same time that Jewish Agency officials were arguing that the fence was "unfortunate but necessary," they knew that there was a steady movement of people going in and out.[32] This movement would mean that from a health perspective, the effectiveness of the quarantine at Shaar Ha'aliya was compromised. Moreover, most Shaar Ha'aliya employees did not actually live on the premises; they commuted every day, which makes it all the more clear that the quarantine at Shaar Ha'aliya was not hermetic. And so the argument being made (that they needed to isolate the people in Shaar Ha'aliya to isolate their diseases) does not make sense.

This, then, raises the question: How could the same people who knew that the quarantine was ineffectual still insist that it was medically necessary? One possible answer is that they were just using the term *quarantine* incorrectly. Shaar Ha'aliya was, in fact, simply a processing camp of which medical exams played a part. This explanation seems to make the story of Shaar Ha'aliya very simple, but it is in fact evasive and superficial. It does not give the nuances and undercurrents of the camp, the mass immigration, and Israel in the 1950s the attention they deserve. And it is the easy way out because it suggests that only people from above—policy makers, public health officials—get to say what is or is not a quarantine. The fuller answer is found in a combination of fear, fences as a meaningful response to fear, and medicine as a powerful conceptual frame.

Fear

In her seminal work on pollution beliefs, Mary Douglas identified foreigners as a group that is "credited with dangerous, uncontrollable powers." They are conceived as a "polluting" and threatening presence and, as a result, "an excuse is given for suppressing them."[33] If we recall, David Musto included the "disease" of immigration in his survey on the various groups that have traditionally been quarantined throughout history. Howard Markel and Alan M. Kraut have both argued that the desire for physical separation from people who are sick is heightened when they are immigrants.[34] Moreover, a central theme in Musto's discussion is a broad idea of the "elemental fear of contagion," which is not purely biological:

> The fear of a disease, as the history of quarantine indicates, arises not
> just from a reflection of the physiological effects of a pathogen, but from
> a consideration of the kind of person and habits which are thought to
> cause or predispose one to the disease.

Likewise, quarantine is a response not only to the actual mode of transmission, but also to a popular demand to establish a boundary between the kind of person so diseased and the respectable people who hope to remain healthy.[35]

When we look to the Israeli setting, we see this combined fear of immigration and disease, blurred boundaries between physical and social contagion, as well as the simple desire to establish a boundary between the "healthy" and the "diseased." It is well-documented that many members of the Yishuv were wary of the mass immigration and the type of people coming in to Israel. Ben-Gurion expressed some of these fears in his journal: "We are facing a wave of immigration that is different from earlier ones not only in its size, but also in its quality. The mass immigration that will now be arriving in the country . . . will mostly be coming from Jewish areas that are materially and spiritually poor . . . the Yishuv's character is at risk of being damaged and its pioneering identity is at risk of disappearing."[36] In his visits to Israel in 1949 and 1950, journalist Irwin Shaw described the environment that accompanied the arrival of the immigrants. After sketching a hectic scene—with the frantic speed of arrival and a mishmash of languages, cultures, and standards of living—he makes it clear that "there is fear" among Israelis that their "conduct and modes of life will be smothered." His conclusion is unsettling: the immigrants "loom as a huge, dark puzzle for a nation rich in puzzles."[37]

Shaw presents the larger, national concern for how the variety of immigrants and their different norms would alter the nation's course. At the same time, he conveys Israeli society's perception of the "dangerous" Moroccan immigrants: "If you stroll about the city after midnight, you are very likely to be approached by the police, who travel in threes, armed with carbines, and who politely remind you that it is not safe to be out so late because of the large number of immigrant North Africans, who have imported into the community their old and unpleasant habit of knife-wielding."[38] In these two passages, the fear of the immigrants is framed both as an abstract apprehension of the influence of the unknown masses as well as a more specific fear of the dark, foreign individual who was perceived as a violent intruder. Moshe Lissak's study on how the Yishuv stereotyped and stigmatized immigrants in this period references these two angles of fear: the quality of individuals and the larger danger posed to the Yishuv's traditions.[39] Shaw's illustration of the knife-wielding North African fits in well with Lissak's study, which shows that the Moroccan immigrants were subjected to the worst, most widespread stereotyping.[40]

We see another depiction of this subject in a passage from Meir Shalev's classic Israeli novel *The Blue Mountain*. During an encounter between a Moroccan immigrant and a veteran (*vatik*)[41] from the mythic Second Aliya, it was explained that the new immigrants brought out the others "scorn and compassion." Shalev describes acts of assistance that were laced with paternalism and contempt. The Israeli villagers volunteered with the immigrants, donated food, taught them skills that would help them acclimate. But then, afterward, when they were alone, the villagers denigrated the same people they had just helped. They spoke of "the little men in blue berets who did nothing but drink, play cards, and shoot craps all day while longing for their caves in Morocco and wiping their rear ends with stones."[42] This example of "scorn and compassion" reinforces the claim that Israelis sympathized with the immigrants while also being suspicious of the changes they were bringing to their familiar world.[43]

But it was not simply a scenario of reservations and hesitations. Ben-Gurion spoke of the "risk" of "damage" and "disappearing." Shaw wrote of the "fear" of being "smothered," and a "looming," "huge," "dark puzzle" while concurrently describing night streets that were not safe because of armed foreigners. Horowitz and Lissak describe "heightened tensions."[44] Henrietta Dahan-Khalev described the Yishuv's "threatened" Zionist identity,[45] while Lissak described "widespread fears and even panic regarding the influence that the immigrants of the 1950's would have."[46]

This general sense of panic ties into the sense of panic that was specific to health and disease that we discussed in chapter 2. The two ideas

being under threat, "xenophobic nationalism," and a desire for exclusion and walling.[59] What Brown is describing beautifully captures the context of Shaar Ha'aliya: a nation feeling vulnerable, with its identity, culture, and economy under "threat" from the "image of immigrant hordes." She describes walling contexts where there is "an increasingly blurred distinction between the inside and outside of the nation itself."[60] She touches on the deep sense of anxiety out of which these walls emerge: "The call for states to close and secure national borders is fueled by populations anxious about everything from their physical security and economic well-being to their psychic sense of 'I' and 'we.'"[61] This echoes back to Moshe Lissak's description of "widespread fears and even panic regarding the influence that the immigrants of the 1950's would have."[62] The immigrants in Shaar Ha'aliya, their religiosity, dress, and culture, were a source of anxiety for many Israelis, a threat of change and difference, a threat of "cultural-religious aggression toward Western values." This was most certainly a case of a nation whose distinction was "blurred," which had a deeply unsettled "psychic sense" of "I" and "we."

This, then, is where walls come in. They symbolize definition where there is confusion, they signify reassurance where there is anxiety, they stage state power where there is, in fact, vulnerability. It is not hard to see how—if Shaar Ha'aliya had been open—it could have given expression to "the nation-state's vulnerability and unboundedness, permeability and violation."[63] Imagine Shaar Ha'aliya without a fence being observed by a Jewish resident from Haifa: newly arrived foreigners, "unbounded," with nothing to stop their visiting family members from coming in and out, nothing to keep the immigrants from flowing into, blending with, the perimeters of the permeable city. This Jewish resident of Haifa would have "the vantage point of a subject made vulnerable by the loss of horizons, order, and identity attending the decline of state sovereignty."[64] We can see how, for him, "amid these losses," of identity, horizons, and order, walls could offer "psychic reassurances or palliatives."[65] And as we imagine a fence being drawn around the camp, we see it defining, containing, to "generate what Heidegger termed a 'reassuring world picture,'"[66] to "express power that is material, visible, centralized, and exerted corporeally through overt force and policing."[67]

Yet Brown is quick to remind us how much of this sense of reassurance is, in fact, a façade: "Walls do not actually accomplish the interdiction fueling and legitimating them."[68] In Robert Frost's classic poem "Mending Walls," the desire to rebel against walls comes from a deep force of nature,

> That sends the frozen-ground-swell under it,
> And spills the upper boulders in the sun;
> And makes gaps even two can pass abreast.[69]

Then why walls? Since there is something to them that deeply engenders rebellion ("Something there is that doesn't love a wall / That wants it down"[70]) and they don't create closure but rather new types of entry, then what purpose do they serve? Brown homes in on the role of performance. Perhaps this is what drew Robert Capa's expert eye to the Shaar Ha'aliya fence: its theatricality. As "spectacle," it projects "an aura" of sovereign power, it projects an image of the state establishing order and control over these immigrants who were, for so many, an unsettling, nebulous threat.[71]

Medicine

In *Discipline and Punish*, Michel Foucault describes quarantine as a "disciplinary mechanism" designed in response to the "real and imaginary . . . disorder" that results from plague. "The plague is met by order; its function is to sort out every possible confusion: that of the disease, which is transmitted when bodies are mixed together; that of the evil, which is increased when fear and death overcome prohibitions. It lays down for each individual his place, his body, his disease and his death."[72] The quarantine at Shaar Ha'aliya was a far cry from the absolute, tyrannical quarantine in plague-ridden seventeenth-century France that Foucault illustrated.

Nonetheless his perspective of quarantine as an attempt to respond to disease with order and discipline ("the disciplinary mechanisms to which the
fear of the plague gave rise"[73]) offers important insight into Shaar Ha'aliya.

There was "real and imaginary" fear among Israelis who felt that their
bodies, lifestyles, and ideals were threatened by the immigrants. Quarantine, that ancient act of separation, has been understood as a means of
self-preservation for thousands of years, clung to as "the immediate salvation of a threatened society."[74] So it was that the Shaar Ha'aliya quarantine was the *perceived* "salvation of a threatened society." Even though the
breaches in the fence clearly show that it did not make sense to insist that a
quarantine was necessary, for those who were feeling threatened, the fence
was a symbol of salvation, comfort, protection, and control. Or as Mary
Douglas has concluded, "I believe that ideas about separating, purifying,
demarcating and punishing transgressions have as their main function to
impose system on an inherently untidy experience."[75]

Yet if it was just an issue of general control, why was there any reference
at all to a quarantine? And why was there such a heavy reliance on the
health rationale to defend Shaar Ha'aliya? In the chapter on Western medical science in the book *Medicine: A History of Healing*, author Ann Dally
has included a section titled "The Rise of Medical Power." This section is
devoted to understanding the exalted position of the medical profession
in twentieth-century Western societies. We see how, through the medical-
ization of domains such as pregnancy and childbirth, contraception, abor-
tion, and drug addiction, medical practitioners have succeeded in "gaining
and increasing its power over many aspects of human life where before it
played no part."[76] Adding to this power is the physicians' privileged knowledge: "They have known secrets, both about poisons and remedies, and
about their individual patients."[77]

But it is not only membership in that elite guild that gave physicians
their authority. The successes of and their connection to biomedicine
gave them even more power and status. In the first half of the twentieth century, scientific medicine could seem invincible, celebrating a "long

anticipated therapeutic revolution."[78] Following numerous successful discoveries, "more than all previous centuries put together" medicine became
"infinitely more powerful than it ever was before."[79] In the first half of the
twentieth century alone, TB (one of the most fatal diseases of the modern
world) was made preventable as of 1924 and increasingly treatable from
1944 to 1956 with the discoveries of streptomycin, para-aminosalisalysic
acid, and isoniazid. In 1921, Frederick Banting and Charles Best's discovery
of insulin dramatically helped turn an often fatal disease into a manage-
able life condition, and Alexander Fleming's discovery of penicillin in 1929
contributed to infection's diminished potency.[80] For medicine, this was
truly "an era of spectacular victories."[81]

Well before the significance of the Nuremberg Doctors' Trial and the
atrocities of the medical system under Nazism were fully comprehended,
this was a period of proliferation of scientific thought and a belief in
the capacity of medical progress.[82] By the time Shaar Ha'aliya opened its
gates, there were precedents throughout the world where state concerns
superseded the freedoms of individuals in the name of the public's health
and under the authority of medical science.[83] Moreover, public health and
medical science were trusted and respected in Zionist thought, as European tools for simultaneously resuscitating the "degenerate" Jewish body
and the "neglected" and "desolate" Jewish homeland.[84]

Shaar Ha'aliya's Israel was born of this context of twentieth-century
medical authority. Although the state had only just been established, there
was already a deep-rooted tradition of medical activity and institutions
that dated back to the prestate Yishuv. When the Shaar Ha'aliya officials
turned to medical explanations, they were relying on a known, trusted,
and prominent authority that made the medical argument seem like the
final, indisputable word. The officials who used the medical rationale
in the defense of the quarantine were themselves part of the environment that was feeling threatened by the foreignness that the immigrants
embodied. As a result, they took refuge in the health rationales they were
espousing. The contradictions between the defense of the quarantine and

the known breeches in the quarantine suggest that the administration's concerns were emotional and visceral fears of foreignness, change, contagion, and chaos expressed in rational, scientifically defensible terms. Mary Douglas has identified this tendency in modern society: "We moderns [. . .] fear pathogenicity transmitted through micro-organisms. Often our justification of our own avoidances through hygiene is sheer fantasy. The difference between us is not that our behavior is grounded on science and theirs on symbolism. Our behavior also carries symbolic meaning."[85] These ideas offer a framework for understanding what was happening in Shaar Ha'aliya: the chaotic environment, the feeling that the absorption of immigrants at Shaar Ha'aliya was spinning out of control, the experience of anxiety, and the reassurance and discomfort caused by the quarantine.

Unfortunately, Sort of, a Quarantine

In March 1951, members of the Labor Zionist party, Mapai, who were stationed at Shaar Ha'aliya drafted a three-page letter to their party headquarters in Tel Aviv.[86] It is a passionate outpouring of deep-rooted frustrations that is divided into two sections: "The Existing Situation at Shaar Ha'aliya" and "The Slander." As a cry from Mapai in Shaar Ha'aliya to Tel Aviv, it illustrates the difficult position the camp's employees were in: they were the ones who had to implement unpopular absorption policies, and they were feeling abandoned by the Yishuv. In the section "The Existing Situation at Shaar Ha'aliya," the authors depict the camp's troubled environment: "The conditions at Shaar Ha'aliya range from difficult to very difficult. The housing conditions are awful, the tents make a terrible impression upon the immigrants . . . the crowding in the camp is very great . . . the mixture of people from all corners of the world, different ethnicities, different languages, different customs . . . all these factors put every immigrant in a bad frame of mind and make them irritable from the first moment they step foot into the camp." This "bad frame of mind" and "irritableness" found a raison d'être in the absorption policy that was geared toward sending the new arrivals to communal agricultural settle-ments (*kibbutzim, moshavim*) or development towns, when most immi-grants wanted to be housed as near as possible to the large cities, particu-larly Tel Aviv and Haifa.[87] The authors describe how this settlement policy made the immigrant "angry with the state, the camp and the institutions." And of course, the most perceptible part of the state, the camp, and its institutions were the absorption workers—the people standing in front of the immigrants telling them where they could or could not live.

The authors are open about the strain that they were under: "The employee is attacked by the immigrant in many different ways, includ-ing curses and physical force . . . the workers in every office toil under incredible pressure from the immigrants." The job's hours, pay, and gen-eral conditions, as described in the Mapai report, only exacerbated their stress: "[The Jewish Agency employees in Shaar Ha'aliya] work overtime with no compensation, they work nights, Sabbaths and holidays. The work itself is quite particular, difficult and irritating, demanding and sometimes dangerous." "The Existing Situation at Shaar Ha'aliya" ends by praising the Shaar Ha'aliya staff while emphasizing how precarious there situation was: "Our work demands incredible mental strength, nerves of steel and dedication . . . the Jewish Agency's system in the camp is working beyond its capacity."

This sense of inundation leads into the fascinating section "The Slander"—half a page of vented frustration and finger-pointing and, ulti-mately, an appeal for assistance. The writing is forthright and accusatory: "And what is [our] reward: slander. And who is doing it? No less than the central agents in Mapai; its newspapers and its people." The authors accuse the critics of Shaar Ha'aliya of making unconstructive attacks that do not offer any solutions but rather undermine the work being done by the absorption workers at Shaar Ha'aliya by "making empty promises to the immigrants." The Mapai authors restate their belief in the Shaar Ha'aliya staff before closing their letter with a barbed appeal: "Join us in fixing the situation and don't dance a demonic dance around us. . . . Help us and don't hinder us."

The dominant themes of this letter are exhaustion and resentment. The picture that crystallizes is of young idealists, who had dreams of "seeing the existing situation and trying to fix it," being bogged down by the realities of implementing a flawed policy upon a hostile crowd. But the issue that seems to have aggravated them the most is that while they were actually doing this demanding work, their party members—the ones who were not there at Shaar Ha'aliya trying to "fix the situation"—were openly criticizing their efforts. It is significant that in the report, the immigrants are also shown to suffer as a result of the absorption policy. The Mapai authors show how the fate of everyone at Shaar Ha'aliya, staff and immigrants alike, is linked:

> [The long lines] sometimes make it impossible for the clerk to properly explain, to those interested, the reasons why their requests were not carried out.
>
> The pioneering roles that the state assigns the immigrant "occasionally against his will" determine the immigrant's approach to the clerk.

This report describes a situation where everyone at Shaar Ha'aliya was suffering at the hands of a flawed and overwhelmed system. By depicting the immigrants and the employees as a form of an alliance, the authors convey a sense of the rest of the country being poised against Shaar Ha'aliya and all its players. This impression is reinforced once again by Weisberger's involvement in the report. The copy found in Weisberger's file is a typed document, presumably the Mapai authors' original, with detailed corrections added in Weisberger's handwriting. This creates a new particular document with interaction between the voices: the uncensored voice of the Mapai representatives, the edited version that merges

Weisberger's voice with that of the original authors, and Weisberger's editorial decisions, which are, in and of themselves, revealing.

The overall change that comes through Weisberger's editing reinforces the authors' claims of the Shaar Ha'aliya staff being overworked,
underpaid, and underappreciated. It still exposes the tension experienced
by the camp personnel while, in keeping with Weisberger's diplomatic tendencies, softens the wording, making it less emotional, and tones down the
accusations made against Mapai. Where the authors write "existing conditions at Shaar Ha'aliya range from difficult to very difficult," Weisberger
tones it down to "camp conditions are not easy." The original authors
claim that the camp's tents made "an awful impression," whereas Weisberger edited it to "a difficult impression."

Weisberger cuts out many sections altogether. What is perhaps most
interesting is his censorship of the first three paragraphs of the section
"The Slander." These paragraphs, the most unleashed criticism of the
Mapai leadership, receive a simple response from Weisberger: they are
crossed out with a large X. But even as he edits with such bluntness, Weisberger still allows the letter's most important claim to come through: the
Yishuv was subjecting the Shaar Ha'aliya staff to unfair criticism.[88]

In this letter, in fact, two texts refer to the quarantine. The original
authors of the letter explain that "Shaar Ha'aliya is a quarantine, transit and processing camp for new immigrants." This point is conveyed
briefly and matter-of-factly, not unlike the way it comes across in the police
documents. It isn't a problem or even a big deal. But then a second voice,
that of Yehuda Weisberger, comes out through his handwritten corrections.
Weisberger changes the statement to read, "Unfortunately, the camp very
quickly became a sort of large quarantine."[89] It is a small alteration, but it
is telling. What is the difference between "a quarantine" and an "unfortunate, unintentional and sort of, large quarantine?" The first is unques-
tioned, deliberate, and definitive: this is just the way it is. The second
is hesitant, regretful, expressing hints of shame and indefiniteness. It is

unfortunate that this is the case. It is not what we would have wanted, and it isn't even *exactly* a quarantine but it, kind of, became one.

The end result is very different from the unapologetic stance that Weisberger took in his 1950 *Jerusalem Post* letter. Part of this is almost certainly an issue of audience and context. In the *Jerusalem Post* letter, he is angry that Shaar Ha'aliya has been attacked. He is defensive, assertive, abrasive, and even nasty. Through the Mapai letter he is—indirectly, via his edits—speaking to his superiors. Throughout the letter, his corrections and changes are consistently mollifying, leaving a far more moderate text than what he was given. This is Weisberger the diplomat at his most diplomatic. His diplomacy may be the result of not wanting to upset his superiors. It may be him acting as a guide (or censor) to the passionate authors of the text. But his revisions show a hint of leeway, a slight acknowledgement that this idea of a quarantine was not without its problems, that it was not necessarily as simple as the "it is a quarantine" that Weisberger had declared so clearly at other times and that the unedited Mapai text suggests so simply and straightforwardly.

A Gate of Immigration or a Quarantine Camp?

Just as Weisberger seems to have been wavering over whether the quarantine was punitive or protective, others were more certain: in March 1951, two different articles were published in Israeli newspapers with strong and opposing positions in this argument. Journalist Refael Sela published an article for the left wing, antiestablishment newspaper *Haolam Hazeh* that covered three large pages with text and stirring photographs, illustrating the difficult conditions of camp life.[90] The entire three pages were framed by a bold border of barbed wire, thick and black, at the top and bottom. The barbed wire was a stark statement that suited the article's title, "A Gate of Immigration or a Quarantine camp?"[91]

Sela's main claim was that Israelis needed to see that Shaar Ha'aliya was more than just a processing camp: it was an important symbol of how the

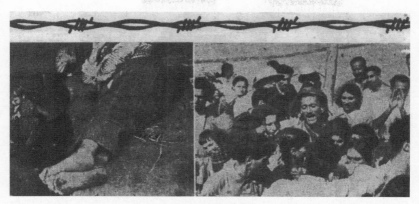

Figure 2. Images of barbed wire and immigrants. *Haolam Hazeh*, March 1951.

new immigrants would be welcomed in Israel, and it was failing. Rather than embracing the immigrants in their new homeland, giving them a warm and eager welcome, the camp's terrible, isolated situation was proof that the "veteran" Israelis did not like nor want the immigrants near them. Sela was careful to point out how hard this situation was also for the people working in the camp: "It is difficult to blame the clerks. They are working in conditions that put human patience to its greatest test." To his mind, the blame was with the Israelis outside of the camp: "In the entire country, in the heart of the regular citizen, the attitude toward the immigrants has changed. The new immigrant has stopped being considered an unfortunate being, the citizen of the future, who should be received with love and help, with the aim of being given full partnership in the country. He has become an annoying, unpleasant problem to be gotten rid of, as soon as possible, by housing him in a transit camp (*ma'abara*) that is as far away as possible, or by hiding him behind a tall wall." He did not disagree that the conditions in the camp were terrible; he bluntly and honestly described the camp's awful conditions. What he said was that the rest of the country was blaming the immigrants for the camp's problems, associating them entirely with this place and all its problems and then trying to cast them, physically and socially, outside of Israeli society. Sela argued that actually Israeli society outside the camp walls, the "veteran" population, was responsible for the "degeneration" of the camp and, by association, the "degeneration" of the new immigrants. "Residents of Haifa claim that the criminal world has gotten a hold of the camp; that girls from the camp fill whore houses. But there is no doubt that the root of evil is the camp itself, which sentences its residents to degeneration and idleness that corrupts their first days in their homeland." This reference to "degeneration" is a subversive term for a Zionist to use as criticism of Israel, and it is repeated throughout Sela's article. "Degeneration" is associated with the Zionist physician and intellectual Max Nordau who used it as a way to describe the physical and social decline of Jewish life outside of the land of Israel.[92] Yes, Shaar Ha'aliya is degenerate, Sela claimed, but it was the rest of Israel that was to blame for this, not the immigrants. "Anyone who sees the conditions in the camp cannot help but think: Zionism is also dead in the State of Israel. Otherwise, there is no possible explanation for new immigrants being received in a camp that forces them to live, for weeks on end, a life of complete degeneration without any form of occupation." The root of the problem for Sela was isolation. Shaar Ha'aliya is a quarantine, he explained. Its isolated location, its barbed wire, and its concrete walls keep the immigrants physically and emotionally cast out of Israeli society. The established Israelis do not want to have anything to do with them. They don't even want to see them, and so they are kept behind walls. The immigrants feel this rejection, and because this is their first "home" in Israel, it taints their entire immigration experience. This theme of the isolating quarantine appears, in text and in images, again and again, throughout the piece. Sela opens the article with a story: "A man peeked out of the windows of the Chrysler that sped past the Shaar Ha'aliya camp, he glanced at the tall concrete wall that straps the camp in like a belt, and spit out: 'It's good that we can't see them anymore!'" It's not clear whether Sela invented this story or whether it actually occurred. But he described this man as a symbol of Israelis, "all the thousands of people" who pass by the camp every day and either give it no thought at all or, like the man in the story, look at it with animosity. One of his most biting comments is an accusation of hypocrisy: "The Yishuv, while pounding away at the drums of the Ingathering of the Exiles—mostly to get itself, and donors from America, all excited—encloses the new immigrants in a quarantine that is surrounded by barbed wire and police and whose tall walls block out a disgraceful situation." Sela finds the imagery of the wall and the barbed wire particularly disturbing: "This is the reception: barbed wire."

If a reader is unmoved by the text and the barbed wire border, the images that accompany the article make apathy practically impossible. The first page of the article has three stirring photographs that capture the main ways that Shaar Ha'aliya makes the people there suffer. The middle of the page has a photograph of an impossibly long winding line, with people of all ages waiting in the sun. There are more than one hundred people in queue. On the bottom of the page, there is a beautiful image of a family resting on the camp beds in an arrangement that is both humble and public. And then, at the top of the page, with a place even above the title of the article and the author's name, is a photograph of Shaar Ha'aliya's barbed wire fence. In this picture, the rolls of barbed wire have been pushed down. A middle-aged woman (she may in fact be elderly) is stepping on the tangled wires. Standing in a manner that looks awkward and unstable, she is being helped by a man on the other side, also seemingly elderly, who is grasping her hand and watching her as she takes a step. This pose of an adult woman in a skirt, moving unsteadily over sharp wires, seems humbling, if not humiliating. And yet there is also room to interpret the action in the photo as empowering, as people saying, "Although we are no longer young and agile, we will not be repressed by an intimidating barrier and we will not be caged." You can't make out the expressions of the couple photographed. We can't tell if they are suffering, angry, irritable, or smiling, joking, or perhaps enjoying their adventure. The focus of the frame is bodies in dialogue with an ugly barrier. Both interpretations fit with the message of Sela's writing: the fence is shameful, the people are not.

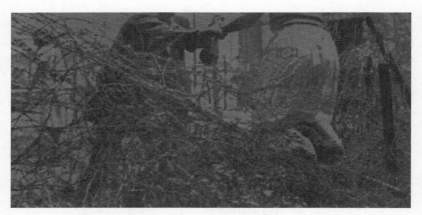

Figure 3. Climbing over barbed wire. *Haolam Hazeh*, March 1951.

The barbed wire appears most prominently in this particular photograph, but it is also the subject of two other pictures that accompany the article. In the middle of the second page there is a small shot of people crawling out through the barbed wire. This is juxtaposed with a photograph of a wall being built to fortify the breached fence. There is a written caption underneath the two:

> "Welcome?" The camp is surrounded by barbed wire. To put an end to
> the breaches a tall wall is now being built [. . .] The administration's
> claim: the immigrants come into town, do dealings on the black mar-
> ket and spread sexually transmitted diseases. But to the world the wall
> looks like a remnant of the regime of Nuri al-Said in Iraq, as a reminder
> of the camps in Eastern Europe. They brought us here for this? They
> complain. The administration's plan—to paint the wall white, to paint
> "Welcome," in spectacular lettering—will not put an end to these com-
> plaints. They don't want the wall.

Sela raises the popular idea that the immigrants' diseases make the isolation necessary. In addition to the reference to sexually transmitted diseases
that appears in the caption under the fence and wall photos, there are two

other references to this theme. One follows the story of the man driving by in the Chrysler: "If we asked the man he would find explanations
for his behavior: the immigrants broke out of the camp to the city, sold
gold watches, cans of meat, sausages on the black market; they bring sexually transmitted diseases into the city (particularly syphilis); they started
knife fights, street fights, outbursts." The next reference comes later in
the article: "The wall can be justified through logical explanations, which
is what Kalman Levin—the dedicated administrator from the Jewish
Agency's Department of Immigrant Absorption—does: fixing the barbed
wire is very expensive, a wall is needed to protect the city from contagious
diseases, also to protect the immigrants themselves." It is not clear what
exactly he means when he says it is "to protect the immigrants themselves,"
perhaps this ties into other claims that "the criminal world has gotten a
hold of the camp" or, later, that there are children in the camp who do not
have parents and are easily preyed upon.

The theme of quarantine preventing the spread of disease appears in
the text several times: "They bring sexually transmitted diseases into the
city," "a wall is needed to protect the city from contagious diseases," and
"the administration's claim: the immigrants come into town, do dealings
on the black market and spread sexually transmitted diseases." For two of
these three references, the camp administration is given as a source, for the
third it is "the man in the Chrysler" that symbol of the apathetic Israeli.
Sela does not seem to dismiss these claims. He attributes them always to
others and frames them as "logical," "rational." However, throughout the
article, he emphasizes that where the country is going wrong, failing
the immigrants and allowing for Shaar Ha'aliya's decline, is by honor-
ing only these logical justifications and ignoring the power of symbols:
"Beyond every argument, beyond every convincing explanation there is a
cancerous truth." He says, yes, "in theory," Shaar Ha'aliya is nothing more
than a processing camp. But he argues that there is much more beyond this
theory: "For the 300,000 immigrants, who have gone through the camp up

until now, this was much more: the first experience in the State of Israel, the first greeting that the country gives them." One symbol he introduces is the camp itself, as a symbol of the immigrant's welcome to the country. The other symbols are the fence and the wall: "But the wall is a symbol that no explanation can negate: a symbol of division between peoples. A symbol that says: the state no longer believes that it can absorb the immigrants by way of the heart. She [the state] has given up her foremost, most holy responsibility: to penetrate into the heart of the person she is bringing to the land." Perhaps the greatest power of this article is that it is one of the few documents (if not the only one) that challenged the finality of the health explanations presented by Shaar Ha'aliya officials. The article raises the issue of the state's moral obligation to the immigrants by asserting that, regardless of the claimed health threat, the state was obligated to embrace the immigrants and that putting them behind imposing barriers was unacceptable. It does not accept the threat of contagion as omnipotent. It proposes that physical contagion is not the only threat to a society: the alienating, isolating symbol of the wall was a threat in its own right. Sela's article is more than a critique. It is an appeal for humanity, compassion, and hospitality. He asks, "Do things have to be this way? Can we not absorb [the immigrants] through the power of love?"

Israel's Gate

Sela's explicit criticism was aimed at the country at large; and as we have seen, he openly expressed sympathy toward the camp's staff. Nonetheless there were people in the Shaar Ha'aliya administration who were upset by this depiction of the institution that they were running. In response, they cooperated on a different article titled "Israel's Gate," which was written by journalist and former Palmach member Pinchas Yorman and illustrated with photographs by Boris Carmi.[93] "Israel's Gate" forcefully challenges and even snidely derides Sela and his thesis. It is not clear who initiated

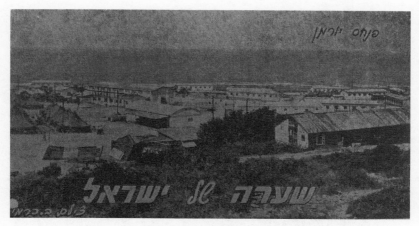

Figure 4. A tranquil image of the camp. Photo by Boris Carmi, 1951.

Yorman's article. It may have been someone in the immediate levels of the camp administration or maybe someone in the Immigration and Absorption Department of the Jewish Agency. Regardless of whose idea it was, there is no question that both Yehuda Weisberger and his deputy, Haim Goldstein, were directly involved in its development. They are both mentioned by name and quoted repeatedly, offering facts and information to help counter Sela's specific claims.

"Israel's Gate" and "The Gate of the Country or a Quarantine?" frame Shaar Ha'aliya so differently it almost seems like they are talking about two different places. While the first article shows photos of crowded lines, people lying on the ground, children playing in dirt, and people maneuvering the barbed wire fence, Yorman's has photos that show order, industry, and tidiness.

The top of the article has a large panorama of the camp site. There are hardly any people around, and the long, orderly huts and view of the sea epitomize calm and structure.[94]

A smaller photo on the second page shows dark-haired men in suits and button-down shirts reading at a table in a clean, modestly decorated room. The caption reads, "In the reading room—a cultured atmosphere."

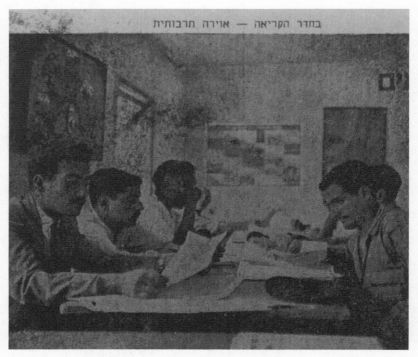

Figure 5. The caption reads, "In the reading room—a cultured atmosphere."
Photo by Boris Carmi, 1951.

Perhaps most significantly, in Yorman's article, there is not a hint of the
wall and barbed wire that were featured so prominently by Sela.

In the middle of the first page, he makes it clear that this article is all
about responding to Sela: "The newspaper Ha-Olam Hazeh (volume 709,
31.5.51) is lying on the camp director's desk. The first pages are devoted
to a sensationalistic article—'A Gate of Immigration or a Quarantine
Camp?'—No less." Yorman makes it known that Sela is a member of
Herut. As a result, his writing is politically motivated and cannot be
trusted, especially since he is collaborating with the radical paper *Haolam Hazeh*: "Well, you can imagine what fruits could be expected to blos-
som out of a connection between a writer from Herut and the editors of

Haolam Hazeh [. . .] The article is so full of distortions that it is hard
to know whether they are the product of malicious intent or complete
ignorance of the subject at hand." With Weisberger and Goldstein's help,
Yorman carefully refutes Sela, point by point. Yorman writes that the camp
did not hold ten thousand people, as Sela had asserted, but only seven
thousand, "according to precise lists from the camp's offices." He asserts
that Sela's description of new immigrants who only had hay to sleep on
(because the material binding the mattress had been removed by previous tenants) was impossible: "To the best of the camp administration's
knowledge," this could never have happened, since "the camp's sanitary
workers go through every tent and every living quarter after the resident
has left and before a new resident arrives, and disinfects the beds and the
mattress." He is lavishly sarcastic about the depiction of Shaar Ha'aliya's
lines: "Mr. Sela made a resounding discovery and he announces it with the
triumphant demeanor of Columbus discovering a new continent [. . .]
It seems to us that also in the State of Israel, outside of Shaar Ha'aliya's
walls, there are lines. Food, the cinema, buses, the Israeli citizen acquires
all these through lines." Yes, there are many lines, Yorman writes, but they
are a part of life everywhere in Israel, and the ones in Shaar Ha'aliya are
the best that they could be under the circumstances: "It is hard to imagine
it possible to have a more productive, quicker method than what I saw in
these lines." Yorman never actually says that the lines are not bad and long
and unpleasant. He just says that the staff are doing their best to keep the
lines moving while still doing their jobs to the best of their ability. And
he completely dismisses the idea that the line is a cause of any suffering
for the immigrant or that in Shaar Ha'aliya, it is uniquely difficult. He
emphasizes the theme that life outside of Shaar Ha'aliya (Tel Aviv is his
go-to reference) is also hard. People in the rest of Israel stand in lines, he
says. Lines in Tel Aviv can also be unpleasant: "In a decent line of Tel Aviv
residents waiting for a movie on Saturday night do not curses fly, heaven
forbid?!"

Yorman's explicit argument is that the Shaar Ha'aliya system and personnel are logical and civilized. His implicit argument is that the immigrants are not. This is encapsulated in his opening story. He describes a
meeting between a clerk who was giving out housing assignments and an
immigrant who wanted to live in Afula near his brother. By the second
line of text, the immigrant (who is never given a name) is identified as
coming from Babylon (i.e., Iraq). "Look," the clerk explains, "Afula isn't
possible. There's no room. But Ginegar is close to Afula. You can see your
brother whenever you want." The immigrant brusquely refuses, "I don't
want Ginegar," and leaves the office. At that point, the immigrant inquires
into Ginegar's exact location from another man outside the office, "a
young Jew wandering aimlessly with nothing to occupy him." The reader
later learns that, unbeknownst to the immigrant, the "young Jew" is a
communist mole, hanging around the camp looking to stir up trouble.
He lies to the immigrant. He goads him, saying that Ginegar is in fact
in southern Israel, far from Afula: "Don't go there. Don't give in. They
want to trick you. They are lying to you." The immigrant takes the bait,
returns to the clerk, and continues to refuse Ginegar even after the clerk
"does not lose his composure, takes out a map and indicates to the immigrant" where it is. The immigrant rips up the map and spits on the clerk
"in a fit of rage." He is joined by backup: "friends, family and just random
immigrants who like violence." In this story, the clerk is extremely patient,
reasonable, and level-headed. The Iraqi immigrant is hot-headed, irrational, violent, impatient, ignorant, and impressionable. It is a depiction that
perfectly embodies the Ashkenazi Yishuv's stereotype of Shaar Ha'aliya's
"Oriental" immigrants.

Yorman is so set on defending his Mapai colleagues against Sela, the
Herut-affiliated author, that his description of Shaar Ha'aliya is utterly
whitewashed. He easily dismisses any claim that might suggest that life
in Shaar Ha'aliya is particularly hard: "The crowding is not terrible." The
conditions are "sparse and simple but by no means are they terrible or

inhuman." He makes repeated parallels to the conditions outside of the Yishuv: The line is normal, just like a line for a movie in Tel Aviv. The immigrants at Shaar Ha'aliya don't sleep in villas but "last I checked not every Jew has a villa on the Carmel."

Whereas Sela puts the fence and quarantine at the top of his article's agenda, Yorman does not; but around half way through "Israel's Gate," Yorman devotes three long paragraphs to a strong and derisive refutation of Sela's argument about the quarantine:

> The honorable author of Herut—Ha-Olam Hazeh objects to the barbed wire fence and concrete wall that surround Shaar Ha'aliya. He admits, however, that this can be explained through logical reasoning: "A wall is needed to protect the city from diseases and to protect the immigrants themselves. However a wall is a symbol of a division between peoples."
>
> Oh how bitterly Mr. Sela weeps.
>
> The simple truth is that Shaar Ha'aliya is an isolation camp (known in other languages as quarantine). That is to say that when the immigrant enters it he must undergo strict medical examinations, including a lung x-ray. If the state of his health is satisfying then he is directed to the processing committee that determines his future place [of residence], and after a week to fifteen days he leaves the camp. However, if it is discovered that the immigrant has any sort of illness—his exit into his new life is put on hold and the immigrant receives the appropriate treatment.

If we look here at what the quarantine means to Yorman, we find logic, reasoning, a "simple truth." It is part of a system of order and authority: strict medical examinations. It is associated with powerful technology: a lung X-ray. He looks at it wholly from the perspective of someone on the outside who does not in the least question the system. For Yorman, it is not messy, not emotional. His parenthesis "(known in other languages as quarantine)" is a subtle and telling reminder that this is not just a system we use here, in the backwaters of small, emergent, provincial Israel. No, what we are doing, this quarantine, is part of something larger, a logic that is known beyond this small place, throughout the world and in other languages. It connects Israel to the world and gives quarantine more authority by association. But there is also something important being conveyed in the way he derides Sela. He is suggesting not only that quarantine is logical and straightforward but that anyone who imagines it otherwise, anyone who does not see that it is "simple," and anyone who sees it as messy, emotional, and upsetting is worthy of scorn and condescension.

Yorman's passage on quarantine continues as follows:

> Now, let's imagine to ourselves that Shaar Ha'aliya were wide open and anyone and everyone would come and go (in accordance with the medical wisdom of Haolam Hazeh). This would mean that an immigrant with active tuberculosis would ride on a busy public bus to Haifa and to any other place. The same with eye diseases, sexually transmitted diseases, etc. This means that the first security measure to insure the extermination of the diseases is the (partial) isolation of the sick immigrant.
>
> Thus the wall which, by the way, is not a tall concrete wall, but rather a low brick wall. . . .
>
> And it is not only because of the health problems that the gates are locked.
>
> The fear is based on profiteering, black market business, theft—all these together are additional factors that motivated the camp administration to act as they have acted.

Here, Yorman introduces fear and the threat of the contagious immigrant. He paints a scary image for his readers of a threatening and anonymous force that could mingle "among us," unbeknownst to us; come into our places, our cities, our buses; and bring harm upon us. This is a defense of the quarantine that would be hard to challenge, since the fear of disease is so visceral and alarming and the image Yorman uses is so accessible. In *Isolation: Places and Practices of Exclusion*, Strange and Bashford have explained this type of approach: "Expounding theories of cure proclaimed the important message that therapeutic practices of isolation were the marks of a civilized society. Exclusion is rationalized in legislation and politicians' speeches but it is also legitimated through appeals to public fears and sentiments concerning suffering."[95] Yorman would have his readers feel that, given the danger the immigrants embody, the "(partial)" isolation and "a low brick wall" are really so little to ask. Again his derision is significant: "In accordance with the medical wisdom of Haolam Hazeh." The implication is that the bleeding hearts know nothing about medicine. If we followed their ignorant advice and if they had their way, the outcome would be disease, harm. We on the outside, in the cities, in Haifa need this barrier for our security. If only temporarily, we need to keep these people away from us. And we do not need to feel bad about the immigrants being isolated in this place. Since, as Yorman and "the facts" have shown, the conditions in Shaar Ha'aliya and the "low brick wall" are not that bad. They are hardly any worse than conditions in Tel Aviv.

His final paragraph about the quarantine brings his earlier defense into question. It also gives a broader expression to the ideas of fear and contagion. If, as Yorman has stated, Shaar Ha'aliya is a medically necessary quarantine, then isn't that enough? Is it not the "simple truth" that he presents earlier? This brief addendum would suggest that it is not quite so simple. It was not only the immigrants' bodies that were sickly and contagious, it was also their morals and their lifestyles, which were threatening to contaminate Israeli society. "Theft," "profiteering," and illegal business practices thus justified incarceration. Throughout "Israel's Gate," Yorman belittles and demonizes the immigrants. Where there are problems the immigrants are to blame. The lines would be more tolerable if the immigrants weren't ignorant: "If the immigrants kept to the appointed time they would save themselves unnecessary waiting. The problem is that not everyone knows how to read." The housing assignments (sending an immigrant to Ginegar rather than Afula) would be pleasant and reasonable if the immigrants were not violent, impressionable, and irrational.

His defense of the quarantine also follows this reasoning: it would not be necessary if the immigrants were not physically and socially tarnished.

Sela wonders whether Shaar Ha'aliya's most important role is as a symbol—of isolation and of the immigrants' poor welcome. Yorman also considers Shaar Ha'aliya's greater meaning, in an early passage: "Is it an immigrant camp? No, it is more than that. Immeasurably more. A boiling cauldron of humanity. A stormy and distraught vessel, a great creation that must overpower impulses. An experimental greenhouse in which east winds blow, scorching sirocco winds and a burning heat wave. Torment and redemption. Light and shadow. White and black." This flowery excerpt gives added insight into the way Yorman interpreted the quarantine. He saw Shaar Ha'aliya as exotic, dramatic, and disembodied. His image of Shaar Ha'aliya did not include any injury to the immigrants. It ignored the specific human experience for the immigrants in Shaar Ha'aliya but not for the workers. In this dramatic, metaphorical passage, the logical, solid solutions offered by the state (vessel, a great creation, greenhouse) are up against the immigrants' pulsing primitiveness (boiling, stormy, east winds, scorching, burning). For Yorman, Shaar Ha'aliya and its quarantine are part of a simple dichotomy of the good and proper (redemption, light, white) up against the degenerate and reprobate (torment, shadow, black).

Shaar Ha'aliya and Modern Policies of Isolation

The conflict over the meaning of Shaar Ha'aliya's quarantine was unsettled and often severe. It touched upon fundamental fears: Now that the Jewish state is finally established, how can we allow it to have any symbols associated with European oppression? Now that that Jewish state is finally established, how can we stop it from being threatened by disease? But not only was there little agreement, the different positions were a wide range of extremes: an imperative security measure, a safeguard, a painful symbol, a prison, a concentration camp. At the heart of this conflict stands the porous yet medically justified barbed wire fence—a simple, powerful and flawed symbol. It was both an expression of and a response to the "near panic" rippling through Israeli society as it faced the mass immigration with its power, inevitable changes, and contagion (both real and imagined). It meant order, control, exclusion, persecution. It was upsetting, reassuring, isolating, and permeable all at once.

At times it seems that the idea of quarantine as a security measure was limited exclusively to people who were responsible for the camp's administration within the Jewish Agency. This leads to the possibility that the protective meaning of quarantine was a PR construction that both began and ended within the Jewish Agency. But then we see that there were cases where this same meaning of quarantine was introduced by people who did not represent the Jewish Agency, such as American journalist Ruth Gruber and then, later, Israeli journalist Refael Sela.

It is important to consider the possibility that the Jewish Agency used the protective idea of quarantine as part of a PR strategy. This is certainly conceivable, since, as we have seen, a recurring theme in their texts presents the fence as unfortunate but necessary. Yet all the while that they were saying that it was necessary to prevent the immigrants' diseases from reaching the rest of the country, the Jewish Agency representatives knew that the fence wasn't fully stopping people from reaching beyond Shaar Ha'aliya, since the immigrants were breaking through the barrier regularly, the rest of the country wasn't actually protected. This could mean that these officials were using the term *quarantine* incorrectly, or we could take it to mean that they were consciously aware that what they were saying was just rhetoric; the fence was a general mechanism of control and the idea of quarantine was simply masking it, making it more palatable to the public. But there is also a strong possibility that these contradictions were unintentional. We can find insight into this, once again, from Mary Douglas: "It is part of our human condition to long for hard lines and clear concepts. When we have them we have to either face the fact that some realities elude them, or else blind ourselves to the inadequacy of the concepts."[96] Maybe the Jewish Agency representatives did push the protective idea of quarantine as a way to defend Shaar Ha'aliya's image. But they could still very well have believed what they themselves were saying. The people making the health/disease argument were part of the environment that was feeling threatened by all that the immigrants embodied. Even when irrational, quarantine and medicine are authoritative recourses. They offer "hard lines and clear concepts," a sense of control, a perceived solution for the change and uncertainty many Israelis felt during the period of the mass immigration.

Moreover, whether or not people believed that the quarantine defense was just rhetoric doesn't change the reality that Shaar Ha'aliya *was* separated by a barbed wire fence; it isolated a feared population during a time of intense and popular fear of contagion. There was a "marking off," a boundary to isolate a "contaminating" population. Not only does this fit into the argument for a "broader applicability" of quarantine; it also reinforces what scholars have been arguing about the blurred boundaries between systems of punishment and isolation. The fact that it is difficult to say with certainty whether the fence was meant just as a general method of control or as a method to control disease reinforces Shaar Ha'aliya's place within modern policies of isolation. For, as articulated by Carolyn Strange and Alison Bashford, "historical practices of correctionalism within prisons and the punitiveness of medical isolation in modern democracies are often difficult to distinguish."[97] It is precisely those blurred boundaries that made the image of Shaar Ha'aliya so upsetting and made the protective meaning of quarantine so significant. The visual similarities between Shaar Ha'aliya's barbed wire exterior and displaced person or concentration camps were immediately apparent, and so "quarantine" offered a reassuring and acceptable way of seeing the same structure.

One way or another, people were moved by Shaar Ha'aliya's fence. Outsiders and insiders—whether international journalists, Jews, gentiles, established Israelis, new immigrants—had their eyes on this place. They were occupied with what the fence meant and what it said about this new country about which so many people were interested. The fence brought out passionate, often angry feelings. It evoked raw imagery and blatant contradictions. Yet most significantly, it brought to the surface a conflict that has yet to be resolved decades later as, over time, signs of Shaar Ha'aliya, its fence, and its entire, rich, difficult history all but disappeared from the contemporary Israeli landscape.

CHAPTER 4

Memory

SEARCHING FOR SHAAR HA'ALIYA

When driving in to Haifa today on the coastal highway, official green signs direct the public to various local neighborhoods: the Carmel Center, Neve David, and Shaar Ha'aliya. After following the signs at the entrance of the city, turning right at the restaurant Maxim, and then taking the road that leads to the Carmel, there is a place marker: a large stone sign in Hebrew, Arabic, and English that reads *Sha'ar Ha'aliyah*. Today this is an unassuming, residential neighborhood. There are large grassy areas, some low apartment buildings, and except for the name, there is no mark of what it once was.

In and around this area are a few memorials, but they don't have anything to do with the historic Shaar Ha'aliya. One is Gan Ofira, "Ofira's Park." The same type of stone sign, with the same font and city of Haifa seal as the Shaar Ha'aliya sign, explain in a few lines that this park is in honor of Ofira Navon who lived from 1936 to 1993: "The wife of the fifth president of the State of Israel. She was very active in promoting the welfare and well-being of children in Israel." Near the beach, there is Hecht Park, named for a former member of the Jewish underground fighting unit, the Etzel, who was born in Belgium and who made significant contributions to Israeli society and the city of Haifa after his immigration to Palestine in

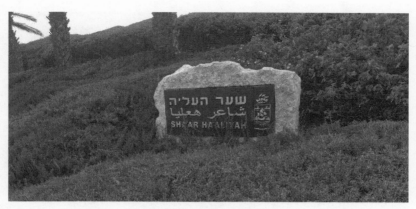

Figure 6. At the entrance of Haifa. © Yaron Pincu.

1936. At the entrance to the park, there is a modest, yet prominent, stone structure that has a photograph of Dr. Hecht and a detailed biography in both Hebrew and English. However, when standing at the memorial for Dr. Hecht, it is possible to see something else: right behind is a sign on which Shaar Ha'aliya appears prominently. It is the local gas station.

Standing here, looking at the gas station, it is almost impossible not to feel that Shaar Ha'aliya has—rather pathetically—been forgotten. To the extent that any memorialization is, in fact, being done at the historic site, it is not for anyone who was involved in Shaar Ha'aliya itself, let alone the immigrants who were there. In this location, which is argu-ably the most symbolic physical spot for the post-1948 mass immigration, passersby can immediately learn about Ofira Navon and Reuven Hecht, but anyone who doesn't know to look for more about Shaar Ha'aliya could just mistake it for any other name on a gas station. Still this is not a complete picture. For one thing, Shaar Ha'aliya does have a place, albeit a small one, in Israeli historiography: it is written about directly in most historiography specific to the period of the mass immigration and in at least one general survey on Israeli history.[1] It is described in music, film, novels, and oral testimony. And while there is no museum where the camp once stood, the neighborhood *is* still officially known as Shaar

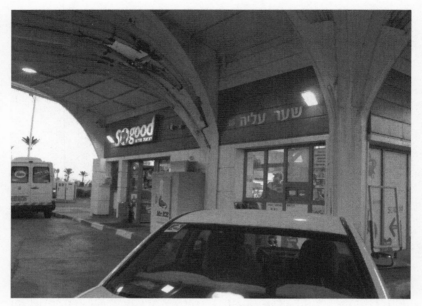

Figure 7. Gas station at Shaar Ha'aliya. © Rhona Seidelman.

Ha'aliya. By leaving the name in place, there remains a trace of—and an invitation to investigate—this past.

This chapter contends with the questions of how and why Shaar Ha'aliya has been forgotten by asking the same questions about the way it is remembered. A beautiful articulation of this dichotomy is found in Yerushalmi's *Zakhor*: "When we say that a people 'remembers' we are really saying that a past has been actively transmitted to the present generation and that this past has been accepted as meaningful. Conversely, a people 'forgets' when the generation that now possesses the past does not convey it to the next, or when the latter rejects what it receives and does not pass it onward, which is to say the same thing."[2] This raises the question: In what ways has Shaar Ha'aliya's past actively been transmitted to the present generation? Has it been accepted as meaningful? Or, conversely, has it been rejected or even not conveyed?

To answer these questions, this chapter begins where there is nothing: the site of the camp. The omission of any historical markers is the most striking example of how Shaar Ha'aliya has been excluded from Israeli national remembrance.[3] To illustrate this point, I compare the absence of memorialization at Shaar Ha'aliya with the abundance of memorialization twenty minutes away at Atlit. Atlit served as a detention camp for illegal Jewish immigrants to British Mandate Palestine. Its heritage site is widely known and hugely elaborate. I argue that Atlit is an important key to understanding why the story of Shaar Ha'aliya has been excluded from Israeli national mythology.[4] Many of the images and themes in Atlit depict the immigrants as victims and heroes, the proto-Israelis as heroes and the British as oppressors, which are some of the exact themes and images in the history of Shaar Ha'aliya: the immigrants are still victims and heroes, but now it is the Israeli state that is in the role of the oppressor. In effect, state-memorialization of Shaar Ha'aliya would be in direct confrontation with the state itself.

This point becomes even sharper through an analysis of the way Shaar Ha'aliya is remembered. Whether in film, song, novels, personal stories, or memoirs, the experience of Shaar Ha'aliya, in all its complexity and variation, is very much alive. And so, following the discussion of the site of memory, I analyze the representation of Shaar Ha'aliya in the rich reservoir of historical remembrances. I argue that these personal remembrances help shed light on why, on an official, national level, it simply is not being conveyed to the next generation.

This chapter uses the general memory of Shaar Ha'aliya as a way to understand the memory of the Shaar Ha'aliya quarantine and vice versa because the two are intertwined. The reasons these are both challenging are the same: an honest confrontation with the memory of Shaar Ha'aliya and its central role in Israeli history would have to include the story of Jewish immigrants to the Jewish state behind medically defended barbed wire. Understanding Shaar Ha'aliya as a quarantine—as implemented and symbolized by barbed wire—is a clue to understanding why the overall memory of the Shaar Ha'aliya processing camp is challenging and currently marginalized.

Sites of Memory: Atlit

Fifteen kilometers south of Shaar Ha'aliya is the Atlit Heritage Site. In its most famous incarnation, Atlit was the location of the British Mandate detention camp for illegal Jewish immigrants to Palestine from 1939 to 1948.[5] Today it is one of Israel's most impressive heritage sites. Before you arrive at the camp museum, there are large, official signs on the highway that let you know you are almost there: Atlit Detention Camp. And these aren't the green direction markers for Shaar Ha'aliya: these are brown guide signs, with a symbol that lets you know you are reaching a location of historical importance. The anticipation is justified. The museum is an evocative and careful recreation of the camp experience. The intention is that you not just learn, but actually feel what it must have been like for the Jewish immigrants who were detained there by the British.[6] They had narrowly escaped genocide in Europe, they were so close to being in the Promised Land but then—right on the shores of the land of Israel—they were detained at Atlit, watched over by armed British guards, and shut behind rows and rows of barbed wire.

Once you are past the parking lot and reception area, you are in the reconstructed camp grounds, which, despite the natural beauty of the place, successfully convey a sense of being contained. The only way to enter the camp is by walking between barbed wire fences. There is a restored watch tower in front of you, a patrol car and two military tanks to your side. A mannequin stands guard in front of a small bus carrying what seems to be newly arriving immigrants with hints of somber faces looking out of the bus's darkened windows. The mannequin that oversees them is dressed as a guard. He is wearing a khaki uniform and has a rifle slung over his arm.

Tours of the site begin in a sparse wooden structure that had once been the registration shack. Visitors then continue in historical footsteps, walking through the premises' expansive, tree-filled grounds to what would have been the next stop for the detainees, a disinfection cabin. You continue on outside and reach the living quarters, a cabin that is brought to life with mannequins set in modest living conditions. There are rows of single metal beds, clothes hanging from rafters, suitcases, wash tubs, a game of checkers to pass the time, and a baby's crib. This is a temporary stop on a migrant's journey. Clearly, it is not the final destination or home, but it isn't an atmosphere of suffering (one of the mannequins is even smiling). It's a setting of tidy simplicity, not squalor. There is a sense of endurance, of making do with an existence that is certainly meager but not deplorable.

The next stop in the tour is the large, restored "illegal immigration" ship. There is a sense of excitement about this ship. The booklet, the website, and the tour guides explain that it was bought in Latvia in 2005 specifically for the Atlit Heritage Site and that it was brought to Israel and to Atlit with great difficulty. It is the most dramatic example of the extensive effort and expense put into this heritage site. It is meant to "perpetuate and commemorate the journey of the *Ma'apilim* [illegal Jewish immigrants] for future generations."[7] Inside there is an elaborate sound and light show that re-creates the immigrants' experiences, the challenges of leaving the only homes they had known, the cramped quarters inside the ship itself, and the joy of arriving at the land of Israel. You come out of the ship's dark, cramped interior and step into the light and fresh air surrounded by green fields. The tour then continues to another cabin to watch a movie that dramatizes the raid by the Palmach, the underground Jewish fighting unit, on Atlit in October 1945, when they liberated all the immigrants who were being detained there. The culmination of the movie is the creation of the State of Israel. An Israeli flag is flown, there is celebration, kissing, and a barbed wire gate opens. With that, the movie ends. This dramatic conclusion to the movie is no accident. Barbed wire is central to the memorialization of Atlit. It appears in photographs.[8] It is emphasized in descriptive texts.[9] It is referred to, repeatedly and with emotion, by the immigrants who are quoted in the museum catalog.[10] And it is physically abundant throughout the camp itself: there is a barbed wire gate you walk through at the entrance of the camp; there are barbed wire fences along the camp's boundaries; and the windows of the registration shack are blocked by barbed wire. In the disinfection hut, there are large photographs of immigrants inside the camp (children and babies, armed guards, people dancing, and others holding large Israeli flags) that span the entire length of two walls. All these photographs are dramatically mounted behind barbed wire.

These images, descriptive signs in the site itself, and the museum pamphlet and booklet make clear that the barbed wire fence at Atlit was callous and repressive. It divided families "with fathers and older children on one side of the fence and mothers and younger children on the other side"[11] and kept the *ma'apilim* from connecting with Israel's beauty: "Here in Atlit, you can no longer see the spectacular view of Mount Carmel that we were so excited to see from the [boat] *Mircea*. Barbed wire fences surround our eyes."[12] The people who are contained inside the camp are

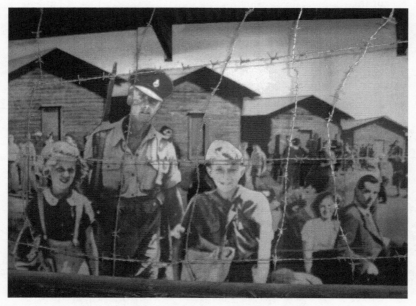

Figure 8. *Barbed Wire*, the Atlit Heritage Site. Photo © Rhona Seidelman.

romantic figures. Although they are victims, they have heroic, valiant spirits that will not be crushed by the fence: "Out of excitement they begin
to dance the *hora* [a traditional Jewish dance] behind the barbed wire
fences."[13] And when they break out of the barbed wire, as part of the 1945
Palmach operation, it is an act of bravery and liberation.[14] Above all, the
Atlit memorialization makes it clear that, of all places in the world, *here*,
this should not have happened to Jews: "After all the hardships they had
endured making their way to Israel, they found themselves once again
incarcerated behind prison bars—this time within the Land of Israel!"[15]
From a Jewish Israeli perspective, the role of barbed wire in Atlit's memorialization is uncomplicated and intentionally emotional. The narrative is
of "us versus them." The British are the oppressors, and the Jews are the
heroes. The British tried to keep the Jews out of the land of Israel, but the
Jews had perseverance, determination, and morality on their side. Then
when the British could not keep these Jews out of the Promised Land, they
kept them captive behind barbed wire.

For this message to be conveyed, the history of Atlit has to be contained.
And as in any history, to keep the frame tidy, certain stories have to be
excluded. In the museum guidebook, you can find hints of events that
have been pushed to the background. One is in the account of the Palmach
evacuation of the camp in October 1945: "When the raid took place all
the *Ma'apilim* were ready to go. Seven immigrants who were suspected of
cooperating with the Nazis were left in the camp hospital, handcuffed."[16]
Who were these men? What happened to them after they were left behind?
It is interesting to imagine how, if told from the perspective of these
shamed, deserted, and suspicious men, the story would be complicated.
Another fleeting allusion that appears in both the heritage site tour and
the museum catalog directly relates to Shaar Ha'aliya. As I was observ-
ing the disinfection hut, the guide pointed out an area in the back: it is a
mikve, a bath for Jewish ritual cleansing. She explained that it was built on
the premises after the state was established. Why there would be people
in Atlit needing a *mikve* after 1948 was left unsaid. As far as the movie

showed it, the state was established, the flag was flown, the barbed wire was cut through, and Atlit was no more. On my tour, this was left unresolved, just another interesting anecdote in a day full of information. For those looking for something of an answer, the guidebook offers this: "The camp was used as one of the first absorption centers for the flood of new immigrants who arrived soon after the founding of the State of Israel."[17] In fact, from 1951 to 1952, the Atlit camp served as Shaar Ha'aliya Bet, the temporary setting to help alleviate crowding at Shaar Ha'aliya.[18] Aside from the *mikve*, there is no reference to this in the heritage site. In some ways, it would then seem that Shaar Ha'aliya has been forgotten twice: once in Haifa and once more in Atlit. Certainly, any historical periodization will, inevitably, leave out some parts of the past. Nevertheless, this double erasure raises the question: What is it about Shaar Ha'aliya that, as yet, just does not seem to fit into the local landscape?

"A Certain Idea" of Israel

The Israeli story, as experienced through Atlit, brings to mind a phrase of Charles de Gaulle's that Pierre Nora confronts in *Lieux de Mémorie*, "a certain idea of France."[19] Nora writes, "Every event on the national scene has brutally and incessantly confronted us as citizens with what de Gaulle, at the beginning of his *Mémoires de guerre*, called 'a certain idea of France.'"[20] This "idea" of De Gaulle's that Nora finds troubling is the harmonious model of France's "greatness and destiny."[21] It is fair to say that there is also "a certain idea of Israel," a similarly harmonious model of Israel's greatness and its destiny that is embodied in the Atlit memorial: Jewish, Ashkenazi *ma'apilim* with an unwavering and unimpeachable connection to the land of Israel face an external oppressor with military bravery, romantic stoicism, heroism, and cunning. And in the end, they are victorious. This is indeed a harmonious model of the past, one that Tamar Katriel has described as nostalgic, heroic, and "sacrifice filled."[22]

It should be expected that official remembrances would be this idealized and this narrow. We know that groups pick and choose their memories and that states use memory to further political agendas.[23] Yerushalmi used a Jewish frame for this universal truth: "For any people there
are certain fundamental elements of the past—historical or mythic, often
a fusion of both—that become 'Torah,' be it oral or written, a teaching
that is canonical, shared, commanding consensus; and only insofar as this
'Torah' becomes 'tradition' does it survive [. . .] Only those moments out
of the past are transmitted that are felt to be formative and exemplary
for the *halakhah* [Jewish Law] of a people as it is lived in the present; the
rest of 'history' falls, one might almost say literally, by the 'wayside.'"[24] For
example, the Torah for pre-1975 France was a glorious history told around
the revolution and the resistance while less flattering histories such as the
revolution's Reign of Terror and the collaborative Vichy regime fell by
the wayside.[25] In Germany, there is a surviving tradition that the outbreak
of World War I was met with collective, "exhilarated patriotism," even
though this was not the case.[26] And while there is little memorialized public history in Toronto, Canada, to the extent that it does exist, it begins
with, and celebrates, British imperialism and colonial markers from
the eighteenth and nineteenth centuries. The history that has fallen by the
wayside is that of the indigenous peoples who have lived in the vicinity of
this city for more than eleven thousand years.[27]

In short, there will always be stories that are forgotten and others, often
whitewashed, that are adopted as "consensus, formative and exemplary."[28]
Not surprisingly, state endorsed remembrances are selected to legitimize
the power of its leaders and ideology and to help shape particular models
of citizenship and patriotism.[29] This is what the Atlit heritage museum
does. As Tamar Katriel has shown, it validates the "Zionist tale" that victimization legitimates the Jewish tie to the land of Israel while also rein-
forcing the central Zionist values of "struggle, choice and human agency."[30]
Through its display of Israel's historic greatness, there is a promise of its

similarly great destiny as the visitors are encouraged to see their own "present and future potential" and to have their "commitment to the national cause" strengthened.[31]

This "certain idea of Israel" engulfs citizens and visitors far beyond what you find at Atlit. In her pioneering work on Israeli collective memory, Yael Zerubavel mapped precisely this phenomenon. In abundant detail, she uncovered the evolution and manipulation of three of Israel's central national myths: the Bar Kokhva Revolt, the Battle of Tel Hai, and the fall of Masada. Through music, literature, folklore, celebrated sites of memory, and state-sanctioned educational material, these historical events have all been transformed into myths that reinforce solidarity, contemporary Israeli political agendas, Zionist ideology, and Zionist interpretation of the past as a way to "actively change the course of Jewish history."[32] This then echoes back to Yerushalmi's words about the histories that are remembered and the histories that are forgotten, since it is no secret that in Israel's process of myth-making many voices were left by the wayside. Those who did not fit into the pioneering, Zionist, heroic mold (such as Arabs, Mizrahim/Sephardim, Holocaust survivors, post-1948 Jewish refugees and immigrants) were excluded. And since Shaar Ha'aliya was the "Atlit" for Mizrahim, Holocaust survivors, and refugees (people excluded from the Israeli myth), the erasure of its historical site is one expression of how the State of Israel has left these people, and their stories, by the wayside. But important distinctions do exist between Shaar Ha'aliya's groups of immigrants and their experiences of absorption in Israeli society. For example, Holocaust survivors were originally perceived in Israel with tremendous derision, but their image underwent a significant metamorphosis, most notably with the Eichmann trial of 1961, when they came to be viewed with growing sympathy.[33] As they and their offspring became an increasingly empowered group in Israeli society, their stories gained a central place in official Israeli remembrance.[34] What has also played an important role, of course, is the fact that remembrance of the Holocaust is a powerful tool in both foreign and domestic Israeli politics. Whatever

the various reasons, the result is that Holocaust survivors and their families have places of remembrance in Israel where their experiences and history are honored and where they are celebrated as essential players in the
state. There is no official state heritage site that does the same thing for
Mizrahim.

However, when we compare the erased history at the site of Shaar
Ha'aliya with the celebrated history at the site of Atlit, it is useful to
consider an idea from Jay Winter and Emmanuel Sivan: "Collective
remembrance [. . .] is rarely what the state tells us to remember."[35] And
indeed, the absence of historical markers at the site of Shaar Ha'aliya is
only one part of the story. Standing in contrast are the vivid, complicated,
and rich memories that are being transmitted through stories, music, and
personal testimony. These remembrances do indeed "demand the right to
be heard."[36] But as we will see, one persistent part of these remembrances
is the image of Shaar Ha'aliya as a fenced-off, isolating space that kept new
immigrants outside of Israel. It is an image that challenges the "certain
idea of Israel."

Shaar Ha'aliya in Art

In *Scapegoat*, Eli Amir's immigration novel set in the 1950s, the young
protagonist, Nuri, is struggling with his identity. As he turns into an Israeli,
he finds himself becoming distanced from his Iraqi immigrant family,
their culture, and their lifestyle. The novel opens with a metaphor for this
change: Nuri leaving Shaar Ha'aliya. He rides a bus up to Haifa as the camp
recedes into the background. Moving slowly up Mt. Carmel, Nuri looks
behind him and sees "a blue sea, far away, and the tents of Shaar Ha'aliya.
Many tents within fences. Like a camp for soldiers who lost the war."[37]
This brief image links Shaar Ha'aliya to conflict, defeat, and confinement.
But Nuri has some release: he is getting away, and Shaar Ha'aliya is behind
him. Haifa is the future, the open, promising ascent into Israel. The camp
is the past—the lowly, fenced-in setting of Diasporic immigrants.

This confining image of Shaar Ha'aliya from *Scapegoat* (1983) is fleshed out by the author in his later novel *The Dove Flyer* (1992). This prequel to *Scapegoat* in Amir's Baghdad trilogy tells the story of how Nuri's family came to flee Iraq, describing the increasingly hostile conditions for Jews that forced them to leave their beloved home. *The Dove Flyer* ends where *Scapegoat* picks up, with the family living in the paltry surroundings of the immigrant transit camp, or *ma'abara*, after spending a few weeks in Shaar Ha'aliya. Amir captures the great disappointment and hardship at the encounter with the camp: "My pregnant mother sat laboriously on the floor of the truck and leaned on the floor, and pulled herself up, and descended and stood and exhaustedly looked upon what was revealed to her. 'Where have you brought me?' [. . .] 'What is the name of this place?' she asked."[38] For the next twenty pages, the harsh conditions in Shaar Ha'aliya are brought to life: filth, spoiled food, despair, encounters with brusque, mocking Israelis and unfriendly new immigrants.

The fence is introduced immediately with the family's arrival at the camp. It is part of the bleak environment, but it doesn't stand out. But then, during their first meal in Shaar Ha'aliya, the youngest son, Moshi, erupts in tears; he is disgusted by the "worm-like" noodles they are given in the camp and hungry for the food he knows from back home: "Moshi turned over his plate and threw it down on the dirt floor and fled from the tent. 'Abed, go get him,' Mother screamed." The mother is consoled by Abed, an acquaintance from Baghdad who had already settled in Israel and was helping the family get adjusted: "Don't worry Um-Kabie, we are in a detention camp, with barbed wire. Where would he run off to?"[39] Even in this moment—when the reader is relieved that the fence could shelter the young child—there is still a sting, with the blunt description of Shaar Ha'aliya as a detention camp surrounded not just by a barrier but by barbed wire.

Later, when the men go to leave the camp for an outing to Haifa, an argument breaks out over how they should go: "Father wanted to go out through the camp's gate and Abed said that they wouldn't let him leave that way. That you have to sneak out through the fence." Abed offered a biting, biblical take on their situation: "You don't understand that you are immigrants in quarantine, tainted, disease-carriers, lice, pestilence, boils, hail, locusts." After an argument, the sons tried to "push and drag" their father through the fence against his will. Abed finds a hole and crawls under with the boys following. When their father still refuses to crawl through, Abed—now outside of the fence—turns to him: "Come. Come and go from slavery into freedom," said Abed. "Isn't that why you came to Israel?"[40] Finally, it is the sea that draws him out, and the scene ends with the father and sons playing giddily, joyfully, in the water and sand.

Scapegoat, Amir's first novel, may in fact be the most wide-reaching, officially sponsored representation of Shaar Ha'aliya known by young Israelis. This classic, short, and accessible text, taught in public schools, is based on Eli Amir's own life story.[41] Born in Baghdad in 1937, he immigrated to Israel in 1950.[42] Amir speaks openly about his own challenges of integration and the discrimination he and his family encountered as immigrants from an Arab country. Whereas in *The Dove Flyer* the reader gets to spend more time with the immigrant's experience of Shaar Ha'aliya and its barbed wire fence, in *Scapegoat*, the reference to Shaar Ha'aliya is fleeting, and it is not continued in the novel. The place where Nuri's family lives is simply an unnamed transit camp. If you are not looking for Shaar Ha'aliya in this text, you could miss it. And yet it is still there, immediately and centrally. The camp fence isn't highlighted, but it too is there. An organic part of the dismal whole, it reinforces the impression that Shaar Ha'aliya and the immigrants who are a part of it are isolated and separate.

Three years after the publication of *Scapegoat*, and six years before *The Dove Flyer*, the famed singer Chava Alberstein came out with the album "The Immigrants," a collaboration with Gideon Hafen, who composed music for the song "Sharalia."[43] Alberstein herself spent time in Shaar Ha'aliya when her family immigrated to Israel from Poland in 1951. She was five years old at the time. By the time "The Immigrants" came out, she had established her reputation as the "Joan Baez of Israel." It was her twenty-eighth album.[44] The song "Sharalia" is a charming depiction of the immigrant encounter with Israel and Shaar Ha'aliya. The music is upbeat, with a tinge of melancholy, and the overall effect is playful. While the lyrics are, on occasion, also playful, they are still a moving, somber account of uprooting. "Sharalia" opens with the immigrants' arrival:

> This story begins at the end.
> A ship with passengers reaches the shore.
> Tired people, in a new land
> stand before a large gate and look upon it in silence.

By beginning "at the end," Alberstein reminds us that the commonly held idea of immigration as a beginning is misleading: there was so much more that happened to these people before they arrived in Israel. There is something somber and immediately isolating about this encounter, as these "tired people" silently gaze at the gate before them. Right from the start, the immigrants are on the outside.

Throughout, the lyrics evoke the immigrants' suffering. Their experiences of the camp are, to a large extent, the familiar challenges of immigration and acclimation. Alberstein describes the people as "tired." In Israel, "nothing is as promised." Their plans prove to be little more than "dreams." They change professions and identities. They struggle with Hebrew, which is described as "hard" and "apathetic," and they crave their mother tongues. Their living conditions at Shaar Ha'aliya are terrible: "roofs fly off in winter," treasured belongings are drenched in rainwater, and "everyone is sobbing." The refrain evokes the immigrants' pain and longing:

> Someone says, "We're here"
> Someone says, "Maybe"
> Someone cries, "We've found it!"
> They whisper to him, "Please God"
> Someone screams, "For now"
> They scream to him, "For how long?"

These are the thoughts of people looking for a home and some peace. Yet what they are experiencing are not only the difficulties of migrants but also the agony and despair of Holocaust survivors. They huddle together, listening to the radio programs that list names of other survivors, hoping to find relatives who have not been murdered. We learn that others don't listen to these programs. In what seems to be a despondent attempt at starting a new life, they have "changed their names." These are people, Alberstein tells us, who have "no more strength" and have "given up."

The camp itself is described as "a grey place with no color, no view." Enclosed by the fence, the immigrants inside have nowhere to go:

On the Sabbath eve we go for a walk.
White shirt, shined shoes.
We go for a walk but there is nothing to see:
A row of huts, a few trees and a fence.
We return slowly, there's no reason to hurry.

The isolation and the fence are subtle images of confinement and disappointment, but no one is actively causing the immigrants' suffering. No one is blamed. The lyrics of this song are profoundly sad, but, at the same time, they are very funny and lighthearted.[45] She takes playful jabs at these immigrants who embellished their pasts, at Israeli bureaucracy, and at the immigrants who cling to that bureaucracy. Overall, if you "visit" Shaar Ha'aliya through Chava Alberstein's song, it's not such a bad place to be. There is discomfort, sadness, and suffering; there is comic relief and tenderness but no anger and no accusations.

Almost twenty years after Alberstein's song first appeared, a wholly different representation of Shaar Ha'aliya came out in the documentary *The Ringworm Children*.[46] As discussed in chapter 1, up until the introduction of antifungal treatment in 1960, the Western medical procedure for ringworm around the world was extremely harsh. Children who underwent treatment were isolated in the Shaar Ha'aliya Institute for Ringworm and Trachoma for one to three months. Their heads were shaved and then waxed to remove any remaining hairs, and then they were irradiated. Physical and emotional scars were an immediate part of this experience. Then in 1974, an Israeli epidemiologist, Baruch Modan, found that the people who had undergone ringworm treatment in the 1950s were at greater risk for head and neck tumors.[47] In 1994, the Knesset (Israeli Parliament) passed the Ringworm Victims Compensation Law, which established that people who had been treated for ringworm in the 1950s were entitled to monetary restitution from the state. Legal proceedings for individuals seeking compensation continue to this day.[48]

For so many people, the bureaucratic machinations of the compensation law as well as—more terribly—cancer and death brought the traumas from the past powerfully into the present. In the early twenty-first century, the testimonies/experiences of people who, as children, were treated for ringworm at Shaar Ha'aliya were brought to a wide public audience in various ways: news broadcasts, internet forums, as well as the 2003 movie *The Ringworm Children*. This movie tells the story of people who were treated for ringworm from 1952 to 1960 at Shaar Ha'aliya. The movie was screened for the first time in 2003 at the Haifa International Film Festival, where it won an award for best documentary. Following the Haifa festival, it was then screened at a select number of theatres throughout Israel. Today it is readily available on various channels of YouTube and has received thousands of views.[49]

Unsurprisingly, the tone of this movie is angry and accusatory, which is immediately clear from the text that sets up the movie's premise: "During the 50's masses of Jewish immigrants immigrated from North Africa. About 100,000 of their children were subjected to X-rays radiation, as a treatment against ringworm. Thousands of them died, and those who survived suffered cancerous after effects. This film endeavors to identify the people who were responsible for this calamity."[50] In the opening scene, a man by the name of David Deeri is filmed traveling to Shaar Ha'aliya for the first time since he was a boy. He speaks to someone off screen:

"Am I nervous?" He asks.

"My stomach is churning. I'm about to go back forty-six years in time, to my long lost childhood, my long lost youth. To relive the event that ruined my life. I remember that the camp was located in the entrance to Haifa, next to the old cemetery."

He continues, saying, "We're talking about seventy thousand victims, most of them dead. Because of that damned concept." As he arrives at a deserted area with old, decrepit buildings, there is a subscript that reads: "Shaar Ha'aliya" Treatment Center, Haifa. At that point, he gets out of the car, looks around and declares, "Here! Yes, this is the place. The sea was over there, and there were no buildings or trees only the mountains at our backs. The train used to run here. I remember how we climbed the fence to watch the trains go by and follow the trucks that unloaded new children, new victims, brought here to be treated so hideously." The movie ends at the same place that it began, with David Deeri in what seems to be the deserted Shaar Ha'aliya, standing behind a wire fence, looking out over the train tracks as the song "The Walk to Caesarea" (popularly known as "Eli Eli") is played in the background.

In this movie, Shaar Ha'aliya is not remembered as a processing camp but only as a treatment center. Anything that this place was beyond the traumatic medical experience does not exist. The physical space shown, the "site" of Shaar Ha'aliya in 2003, is one of decay. This idea is pushed further by juxtaposing it, in images and in words, with an "old cemetery." It is remembered as a place where innocent children were victims, enclosed behind fences, and treated "hideously."

The word *konseptziya* that Deeri uses is loaded with meaning in the Israeli context.[51] It conjures the 1973 Agranat Commission on the Yom Kippur War on the failings and the hubris of the military elite. This word evokes the tragedies that befell Israel because of myopic power. Moreover, even in this short scene, there is an abundant use of Holocaust imagery, with the trains and trucks that unloaded new children, the term *transports*, and Hana Szenes's song "The Walk to Caesarea." This is not only a way to fiercely accuse the Jewish state, it is also a way for people whose stories have been marginalized to claim access to the most hallowed of Jewish/Israeli Ashkenazi traumas. In *The Ringworm Children*, the memory of Shaar Ha'aliya is unambiguous. The harshest ideas are used to convey persecution, death, abuse of power, and victimization. The Mizrahi immigrants are victims who suffer terribly. The State of Israel, its Ashkenazi leaders, and its Ashkenazi medical establishment are the victimizers.

This movie is important because it has given a far-reaching stage to people whose voices had been sidelined. Before the film's release, the public story about ringworm at Shaar Ha'aliya was being told exclusively by doctors, journalists, and politicians. Through this film, we hear about ringworm treatment and all its terrible repercussions by the people who actually experienced it and who, up until then, were not being widely heard. But *The Ringworm Children* is also very problematic—so much so that in a popular news program broadcast in Israel in the winter of 2018, David Belahsan, the filmmaker behind *The Ringworm Children*, denounced his own film. In this television special devoted to the ringworm controversy, Belahsan explains that the movie was not sufficiently developed in its treatment of this highly sensitive subject and that he came out with it too early, and as a result, he concludes that it is negligent and mistaken.[52] The film's problems are indeed severe. It is framed as a documentary, yet it has glaring historical inaccuracies. For example, it claims that one hundred thousand children received radiation treatment, and David Deeri said that seventy thousand people were dead. In fact, around twelve thousand children were treated at the Shaar Ha'aliya Institute for the Treatment of Ringworm and Trachoma. This number includes treatment for trachoma as well as ringworm.[53] The film suggests that the children were intentionally harmed when the existing evidence suggests that they were the victims of a terribly misguided but internationally accepted and common medical procedure. And I strongly believe that the site that the filmmakers show David Deeri confronting was not actually Shaar Ha'aliya. Shortly after the movie came out, I scoured the area of Shaar Ha'aliya, thinking that I would find the old huts that appear in the film. I had with me an archival map of the camp boundaries as well as a contemporary map of the city of Haifa. I found no indication of decayed buildings nor newly constructed buildings that may have, recently, been built in their place. These structures might be near, but they are unlikely the actual "'Shaar Ha'aliya' Treatment Center" as the movie claims. Perhaps the trauma of the place has distorted the memory. Or perhaps the remembrance has been distorted to express the trauma. It is hard to say.

Even though I am aware of this movie's serious faults, I continue to return to it as a consequential document. Charbonneau beautifully describes the value of illness memoirs in a way that, to my mind, also explains the value of *The Ringworm Children*'s imperfect depiction of history: "Memoirs are therefore not documents that make it possible to retrace an improbable truth of history, but monuments erected in honour of the individual, subjective and irreplaceable life of men and women whom the trial of contagion, when it took place, modified in their very flesh and in that body of writing that is their work."[54] The experience of ringworm in Shaar Ha'aliya modified the flesh, lives, and stories of many people. This movie, with all its many grave faults, is a monument in their honor.

In each of these four texts, there is, at the very least, a sadness associated with Shaar Ha'aliya, a bleakness. These are far from idealized homecomings. Alberstein's Shaar Ha'aliya, somewhat nostalgic and romantic, is the most pleasant. Yet this story of immigration is not a grand, heroic voyage, such as, for example, the one conveyed in Edith Piaf's booming rendition of *Exodus*. Nor is it a glorified, jingoistic depiction of the absorbing country, such as the one found in Neil Diamond's "America": "Never looking back again / They're coming to America [. . .] / Home, to a new and a shiny place [...] / Freedom's light burning warm [...]." Admittedly, both of these examples are from different contexts and by artists with less direct ties to the experience about which they are singing. Nevertheless, they help to illuminate what "Sharalia" *isn't*. The experiences and the people in Alberstein's song are small, human, drudging, heartbreaking, aching, and funny. Their immigration is not bombastic and glorious, it is wracked with doubt and stumbles.

Perhaps the main difference between Alberstein's Shaar Ha'aliya and that of the two others is, in fact, humor. Thirty-five years after her arrival in Israel, she was able to look back and see lightness among the struggles. A key to this different retrospective is very likely what came after, or as an Israeli scholar once commented, the answer is in the names.[55] Alberstein is clearly Ashkenazi. Deeri is clearly Moroccan. It is not surprising that the memories of the Iraqi and Moroccan immigrants are colored by the discrimination these groups have experienced in Israel. It must be acknowledged that Alberstein's milieu of Holocaust survivors, as described in "Sharalia," also encountered discrimination.[56] The author Aharon Appelfeld has poignantly described the prejudice that survivors faced and which he, as a young Holocaust survivor, internalized: "They were called 'the Desert Generation,' or 'the dregs of humanity.' Survivors embodied the nakedness of exile, the wanderings, the Holocaust. Like many others, I also did not wish to belong to them, to speak their language, or to be linked to their memories."[57] However, historian Hana Yablonka has shown that, ultimately, Holocaust survivors were rapidly and positively integrated into Israeli society, notwithstanding the emotional, psychological, physical, and social struggles that profoundly shaped this process. Moreover, Alberstein's personal history in Israel is one of brilliant acclaim. And while she herself is openly critical of Israeli policies, including the repression of the Yiddish language and Yiddish culture that were so dear to her home, her success developed out of a trajectory that can be described as predominantly Ashkenazi Israeli conformity.[58] Thus it is not surprising that, when in "Sharalia" she looks back at her first steps in Israel, she is not angry and, although occasionally sad, can still be nostalgic and amused.

In contrast, Eli Amir has said that he began writing as a response to discrimination:

> I think I started to write because of pain. Because of insult. The pain of my father [...] who lost his crown and became a shadow of himself. And the second thing was that at the Hebrew University I felt, as a Jew who comes from a Moslem country, I felt an outsider [sic] I felt, even, discriminated against. [...] I felt that I am, I don't know exactly the term to use, a type of second class human being. And when I was a student I thought: how can I change the attitude toward me and my culture? [...] And so one day I thought, maybe I'll write a story.[59]

The result was his first novel, *Scapegoat*. Appropriately, from this wellspring of insult and pain, Shaar Ha'aliya is recalled without Alberstein's humor.

Yet the role of discrimination in the shaping of these memories is most obviously relevant to *The Ringworm Children*. The gravity of this movie stems from what could be understood as a double injury: the emotional injury that came of discrimination and the physical injury of the aggressive and ill-fated medical procedure. This brings to mind the words attributed to God in *Ritzato shel Haoleh Danino*. This iconic song about the Ashkenazi establishment's poor treatment of Moroccan immigrants as part of the selective immigration policy was written as a biting social commentary by the Ashkenazi poet laureate Natan Alterman in 1955. It was then given new breadth when the Moroccan-born Israeli musician Shlomo Bar put it to music in 1985. In the song, the "Immigrant Danino" stands before a medical selection committee that will determine whether he is physically fit to immigrate to Israel. When they suspect that he has a limp, they ask him to jump. God speaks to Danino, who has been demeaned in front of his children, and makes a promise: "Fear not. I will cover your defect. But

I will not cover up the insult of your people's rebirth, whose light shines in your tears."[60] The "insult" of Israel's rebirth similarly reverberates in *The Ringworm Children* and its remembrance of Shaar Ha'aliya.

In all four of these very different texts the fence is remembered and, by its very nature, it is containing and isolating. Only *The Dove Flyer* calls attention to the barbed wire, but then there is a glimmer of goodness, since its menacing presence is what would keep the boy Moshi from getting lost outside. The idea of the fence that is conveyed in the movie is similar to what comes across in *Scapegoat*, *The Dove Flyer*, and "Sharalia" but far more fierce. In those other texts, the Shaar Ha'aliya fence keeps the immigrants temporarily confined, whereas in the movie, it keeps the children captive.

There is another indirect but very important way that *The Ringworm Children* shapes the memory of the Shaar Ha'aliya quarantine: it not only challenges the "certain idea" of Israel, it challenges the "certain idea" of Israeli medicine. The Jewish Agency took considerable pride in the ringworm campaign, which they expressed through many public displays of confidence in their work. They made presentations about its achievements in congresses.[61] They wrote letters about it to donors from abroad, where it was described as a way to "cure" Mizrahi children and turn them into healthy Israelis. "You may have heard of the latest addition to the camp . . . ," Weisberger wrote to an American Jewish woman who had sent a package to Shaar Ha'aliya and wanted to know how she could help, "a hospital for 500 children established with a view to cure the aliyah of children from Algiers; Tunis and Perisa, arriving here at the rate of a few hundred at a time and invariably infested with Trychophitia or Trachoma both diseases prevalent in those countries and, if attended to in time, leave no mark on the health of the future generation of Israel."[62] They invited the press on guided tours of the premises that resulted in largely laudatory articles.[63] One journalist praised "the blessed activity of the Jewish Agency's absorption department."[64] Another described how the children "learn to value the treatment they are given."[65]

Ringworm was on track to become the Zionist health campaign of the new state, the grand, mythic "success" story that malaria and trachoma had been for the prestate Yishuv. It was a project that could offer pride on a national—and even on an international—level in its application of scientific knowledge and technological progress for the betterment of unfortunate children. It was seen as the best of western health care being given, for free, to children who, were it not for the State of Israel, would have been deprived. It was seen as Jews taking care of their brethren. But *The Ringworm Children* helps show that beneath this eager commitment to and belief in the medical campaign, lie other less heroic undercurrents. The undercurrent of paternalism used ill health as an opportunity to shape children into particular models of citizenship. Irrational anxiety saw children afflicted with a superficial infection as a threat to the greater society. Questionable judgment aggressively applied a medical treatment that had adverse physical and psychological effects on immigrant children, and obeisance to medical authority prevented reconsideration even when the method of treatment was discernibly severe.

The tragic outcome, as conveyed in the movie, was not simply about the failure of any old health campaign. More than any of the other diseases treated at Shaar Ha'aliya, ringworm treatment was put on a pedestal as a symbol of the greatness that Zionist medicine could achieve. The same way that the State of Israel was bringing to life Herzl's dream of a Jewish state, the ringworm campaign was bringing to life his dream of how the Jewish state's biomedical genius and benevolence would bring it glory: "The blessings emanating from our medical institutions, like a beneficial stream, have made more friends for us here in Palestine . . . than all our technical and industrial innovations."[66] However, Herzl overlooked biomedicine's potential for devastating mistakes. As David Musto put it, "the history of medicine . . . is filled with useless and even harmful remedies applied with confidence to the trusting patient."[67] Since the ringworm campaign was placed on so high a pedestal, it had even farther to fall. And fall it did. The subject of ringworm treatment is a wound that is far from healed. In 2017, *The Ancestral Sin*, an Israeli documentary series about the discrimination of Moroccan immigrants to Israel in the 1950s and 1960s, was met with an uproar. One of the outcomes are campaigns to change the names of any public streets and institutions that are named after Dr. Giora Josephtal and Dr. Chaim Sheba, who played leading roles in the establishment of the Shaar Ha'aliya Ringworm and Trachoma Institute.[68] *The Ringworm Children* was the first public memorialization of the celebrated campaign's tragic failure from the perspective of the immigrants themselves. This important remembrance of the patients' experiences of medicine at Shaar Ha'aliya is pained, angry, and accusatory. It is a reminder that when the fear of contagion and the fear of immigrants come together the outcome is sometimes terrible.

Personal Testimonies: Immigrant Voices

In his memoir, *Call It Dreaming*, the acclaimed translator and scholar of Arabic literature Sasson Somekh writes about his arrival and two week stay at Shaar Ha'aliya. He paints a picture of general hardship: endless lines, unpleasant food, and poor living conditions. But what made the setting particularly bad, according to Somekh, was that it was in Israel. For so many of the immigrants, this reception challenged their ideals of what Israel represented. They had expected that in "their own" country things would be different, somehow better and more, than where they were coming from: "But the complaint and the discomfort began to gnaw at the marrow of joie de vivre that characterized so many of them [immigrants at Shaar Ha'aliya], with their hope that they were moving to their own country where no one could demean them because of their religion. Now bitterness spread."[69] This bitterness that Somekh describes is evident throughout personal remembrances of Shaar Ha'aliya. Many immigrants made it very clear that Shaar Ha'aliya was a pitiful welcome to the Jewish state. One immigrant from Bulgaria recalled that coming to Shaar Ha'aliya was a "shock" and that it was lodged in his memory as the worst part of his immigration experience.[70] Many people vividly remember the filth, chaos, and discomfort of their time there.[71] Some describe being disheartened when their expectations and excitement about arriving in Israel were dashed at the sight of Shaar Ha'aliya.[72] One man explained that regardless of expectations and regardless of the fact that it was temporary, Shaar Ha'aliya was simply "awful," a sentiment that many others echo.[73]

However, there are people who have beautiful memories of their time in Shaar Ha'aliya. Corina immigrated to Israel from Romania in 1950, when she was twenty years old. As she stretched out in the sun on a bed in front of a cabin, life in Israel seemed to her to be absolutely wonderful.[74] Sami stayed in Shaar Ha'aliya for two weeks when he emigrated from Iraq in the winter of 1950. He was sixteen years old, without his parents, and having a ball with his friends. He loved the jam, bread, and olives that they would bring back to their tent to eat. During his medical exam, he spoke in Hebrew, and when they weren't able to understand something that the health care workers said, he and his friends turned to each other for help and figured it out. He experienced Shaar Ha'aliya as a fun, liberating adventure.[75]

There are others for whom the stay at Shaar Ha'aliya had little impact. In the scheme of their lives and memories of their immigration, Shaar Ha'aliya played an uneventful role. In an interview conducted in 1990, one man makes only two brief references to Shaar Ha'aliya. The first statement relates to his own experience there:

Q. Where did you arrive in Israel?
A. At Shaar Ha'aliya. From Shaar Ha'aliya I went to Pardes Hana.[76]

The second statement is a general comment about immigration policy in the 1950s: "I explained to him that the immigrants who came from Islamic countries were concentrated at Shaar Ha'aliya, from there they were either transferred to Beer-Sheva in an open truck or were dumped in a maabara to be labourers."[77] In a thirty-seven page interview that focuses on immigration in the 1950s and his own later work counseling and aiding immigrants, these are the only two references he makes to Shaar Ha'aliya. This man was born in Basra and immigrated to Israel at the age of thirty, so he wasn't a child who was shielded from difficulties by his parents. He was from the "marked" group of Iraqi immigrants who, in the eyes of Shaar Ha'aliya officials, were largely perceived as troublemakers.[78] Therefore his apparently easy experience at Shaar Ha'aliya cannot be explained as him coming from a "preferred" country of origin. Moreover, his immigration was in 1950, one of the two most chaotic, overcrowded years in Shaar Ha'aliya's history. Yet despite these factors that could have been expected to have a negative impact on his experience, all he had to say about Shaar Ha'aliya was that he was there.

One immigrant from Azerbaijan remembers staying in Shaar Ha'aliya for around two months in 1951 (a long stay during yet another one of the camp's two most difficult years); his only comment was that it was "not bad."[79] Another immigrant from Libya stayed in Shaar Ha'aliya for a week in July 1949, when he was already a thirty-eight-year-old man. In an interview on his immigration experience, he briefly mentions it only once, saying, "I was there for a week, and then they transferred us to Beer Yaakov."[80] This offhand attitude appears in another interview with a Moroccan immigrant who moved to Israel at age sixteen. He remembers that when he arrived in Israel he was completely alone, but this memory does not seem to have negatively affected his outlook on Shaar Ha'aliya, which comes across as a very marginal experience for him: "They dropped me off at that 'aliya' camp in Haifa, but I have nobody, alone, no family, nothing, later they said to me: Let's move to Beer-Yaakov, there's an immigrant camp there and you'll be happy there."[81] The distance from the immediacy of the events makes these personal testimonies "reconstructed experience, a melding of memory and later elaboration."[82] Naturally, they are shaped not only by what happened at the time but by who the people later became and the issues that became important to their stories and their worlds. To some extent, the range of memories about Shaar Ha'aliya also exists in the specific memories of the quarantine but with more polarization. Most people who remember their experiences at Shaar Ha'aliya, whether neutral or negative, don't mention the fence at all. Two examples of people who do remember the fence, as we recall from chapter 2, were Sylvia and Eliezer Meltzer. Yet Sylvia's prevailing memory of her arrival in Israel, which was also her arrival in Shaar Ha'aliya, is that it was "like a dream come true."[83] And it's not that the fence doesn't factor into her story at all. Not only does she remember it, but it is a central player in her brief Shaar Ha'aliya narrative. Yet it is significant to point out that this memory is not negative. She isn't shocked about being faced with barbed wire and she doesn't dwell on—which gives the impression that she is not upset by—her own statement that "I don't think they let people go out." Clearly, the image of the quarantine is not an obstacle for her, and neither was the structure itself: "I would go out through a hole in the fence," "My uncle used to go in through the hole in the fence," "We used to leave from there," "I always entered and exited through a hole in the fence." For Sylvia and Eliezer, like so many of the immigrants at Shaar Ha'aliya, the fence and going through the hole in the fence were matter-of-fact. Whether going in or going out, this act wasn't hidden, it wasn't a cause for concern, it wasn't oppressive, and it wasn't hard—it was just done.

However, two other immigrants who do remember the fence describe it in extremely negative terms. Yaacov Steiner was twenty years old when his family decided that they would leave Hungary and immigrate to Palestine. He remembers that they made their decision in 1947, on the day of the dramatic partition vote by the UN Security Council, when Jews throughout the world celebrated the internationally accepted plan to establish a Jewish state. It would take another two difficult years before Yaacov was able to realize that dream to "make aliya" to leave behind the world he knew, move to the distant and foreign Middle East, and become a part of the historic creation of the Jewish state. Finally, in 1949, he reached what was now the sovereign State of Israel. He was alone. He had come to lay the groundwork for his family's arrival and to begin his new life.

As chance would have it, Yaacov's immigration took place a few months after Israel had opened Shaar Ha'aliya. For Yaacov, like the majority of the immigrants, it had been so hard to get to Israel. And his idea of "aliya" was full of such hope and expectation of belonging. But when he saw Shaar Ha'aliya, all the excitement that had surrounded this long-anticipated arrival came crashing down. The sight of the camp, its paucity and overcrowding, left him "in shock," but what upset him most of all was that he wasn't allowed to leave: "The real shock came when [my friend] and I wanted to go for a walk in Haifa, and we wanted to leave Shaar Ha'aliya and the camp was closed in with a sharp barbed wire fence [. . .] They simply refused to let us leave."[84] The explanation that Steiner was given was that he was in a transit camp,[85] but he found this perplexing: "I didn't understand where I was in transit to. I thought I was moving from bondage to freedom, from a country where I was a second, third or even fourth class citizen, or even lower, and I was coming to my country." Much like Eli Amir's Nuri, Steiner offers the lonely image of Haifa, the established, Israeli city that was in the distance, out of reach to him while he was behind barbed wire in Shaar Ha'aliya: "I saw the lights of Haifa from the camp and they didn't let me leave."[86]

Mia Abramov remembers having a similar reaction. She was twenty-four when she immigrated to Israel in 1951. Like Yaacov Steiner, she and her family had to wait several years and overcome many obstacles before it was possible for them to leave Europe. There had been such a buildup that her arrival in Israel was euphoric: "From the moment I descended [from the boat] I knew that I had made aliya to Israel, and there are no words to describe [how that felt]."[87] Although her trip had been frightening, the fear passed the minute she arrived: "I felt the relief of freedom. There's nothing more to say. It was a feeling of freedom." Then in contrast to these exuberant emotions, the sight of Shaar Ha'aliya and its fence was dramatically disappointing: "Everything was a blur. It was a shock to see such a thing, with a fence like this in the country that I was ascending to in freedom." She couldn't comprehend that she was expected to be behind barbed wire: "That I would enter a fence like this was incomprehensible." Mia Abramov remembers feeling that, finally, she was living as a free person in her own country and that no one had any business putting her behind barbed wire. Both Yaacov and Mia tell their story of immigrating to Israel with memories of emotional anticipation, as expressed by Steiner: "When I saw the shores [. . .] I was intoxicated by the sight." But this anticipation made his encounter with the Shaar Ha'aliya quarantine even harder. The disappointment can still be felt decades later as Steiner tries to verbalize his disappointment and the struggle to reconcile his "great expectations" with being "greeted by these things." This dissonance between the beauty of their expectations and the bleakness of what they found made Shaar Ha'aliya an even harder pill to swallow. Steiner and Abramov's narratives are of the Jewish immigrant who had to overcome years of obstacles and anticipation before being allowed to immigrate to Israel or "make aliya." And then, when they did finally manage to get to "their own" country, the fence at Shaar Ha'aliya was a disheartening and alienating reality.

Personal Testimonies: Administrators

These many different remembrances of Shaar Ha'aliya are, appropriately, all from the viewpoint of the many immigrants. Two additional texts give the perspective of men who oversaw the camp administration and immigrant health services. *Shaar Ha'aliya: The Diary of the Mass Aliya, 1947–1957* by Yehuda Weisberger is not actually his memoir, although that is how it first seems. While working as Shaar Ha'aliya's director, Weisberger always had a sense of its historical importance, and he set out to write its story.[88] In 1963, several years after he had moved on to a new job, he contacted publishers, writing that he expected his book on the camp to be ready for publication around two years later, in 1965. This goal was still not realized when Weisberger died in 1979. In an attempt to see his work completed, Weisberger's wife, Leah, worked in coordination with friends to publish the 1985 book *Shaar Ha'aliya: The Diary of the Mass Aliya, 1947–1957*. Although he clearly is not the actual author of the book, Weisberger is presented as such, presumably because the contents come from the diary and files that he himself had written and collected. It is not clear who actually authored or edited the manuscript. It is also not always clear when Weisberger's voice ends and where it is the voice of others. As such, it is important to approach this as the complicated source that it is. It is not a primary source because it has been edited many years after the fact by peopled distanced from the actual events. Neither is it Yehuda Weisberger's memoir, even though it is attributed to him. What is certainly clear is that this is a very important book, most obviously because it is the most comprehensive, published manuscript on Weisberger's experience in Shaar Ha'aliya and it is a main source of information on this chapter of Israeli history.[89]

The Diary of the Mass Aliya begins with Yehuda's biography. It then presents the situation for immigrants in Israel during the mass immigration before discussing Weisberger's work as the head of the immigrant absorption center Neve Haim and then his job as the director of Shaar Ha'aliya from 1949 to 1957.[90] Not surprisingly, the perspective on, and image of, Shaar Ha'aliya that comes through in this book are very similar to what comes through in Weisberger's archives. He depicts the many problems that exist in all corners of the camp, whether with the staff or with the immigrants, conflicts between the immigrants and the guards, overcrowding and wasted food. This book gives the administrator's story. It presents the actions and frustrations of a person with good intentions facing an exciting but also relentless, overwhelming task. Weisberger wasn't a high-powered decision-maker; he was the person on site, tasked with the difficult job of seeing Shaar Ha'aliya through the day-to-day. In the book, he comes across as someone working to maintain his position of authority as he envisions it.[91] Perhaps because this book was completed by Yehuda's loved ones, at times, he is depicted as a classic hero: possessing a strong character, persevering, rising to meet difficult challenges. But what also comes through are his own prejudices and limitations, as he looks on some immigrants with respect and others with disdain.[92]

There are not many references to the barbed wire fence in this book. One is part of a broad description of the difficult conditions, such as the long lines, the police guard, the cramped quarters and the barbed wire fence.[93] But there are two other references—one direct and one indirect—that are more complicated. On page 71, in the book's earliest descriptions of Shaar Ha'aliya, it is explained that the Jewish Agency's decision to enclose the camp with barbed wire and a police force was financial: they were concerned that if the border wasn't closed by a fence, then immigrants would smuggle property through without paying taxes.[94] A page earlier, the section on Shaar Ha'aliya opens with a description of the considerations that led to the establishment of Shaar Ha'aliya. The list of reasons—the immigrants posed health risks, were a security risk, were at risk of dodging the draft—are well-suited to the needs of a general immigration processing camp. But in the book, there is no direct suggestion that the fence was because of medical reasons, only economics. This point brings us back to the problematics of this book as a source. This issue, of immigration and smuggling and Israel's early economy, was central to the policy of the mass immigration and immigration processing. However, as a stand-alone explanation for Shaar Ha'aliya's barbed wire fence, this claim contradicts Weisberger's own archival records and the many complicated references to health and quarantine that he himself made to defend and explain the barbed wire fence.

How, then, should this source be approached? And what does it offer? *Shaar Ha'aliya: The Diary of the Mass Aliya, 1947–1957* has been crucial to the remembrance of Shaar Ha'aliya, particularly in historiography.[95] Weisberger's book has been one of the most important sources on Shaar

his beautiful dream of the Promised Land with the dank, grey structures facing him. A five-year-old girl, Hava Alberstein, or Hava Alberstein–like, is shielded by exhausted parents. Frigid, demoralizing, destructive rain is falling into their tent, and they have put an umbrella over their young daughter. They are trying to keep their child safe and healthy, although there is so much working against them. David Deeri, a young boy alone, is there—newly arrived and immediately separated from his parents. His head is shaved and then, painfully and seemingly without reason, it is waxed. Yehuda Weisberger, a young man, newly orphaned by the Holocaust, walks around the camp, trying to maintain control and humanity in an environment that quickly must have felt beyond his control. And then there is Avraham Sternberg who, scanning the sights around him, is envisioning how much worse it would become if an epidemic broke out. Faithfully, perhaps desperately, perhaps even blindly, he turns to medicine as a solution for control. All around are the tents, the lines, the strained encounters between people. And of course, there is the fence, containing, or trying to contain, it all.

These vivid images bring back the earlier questions of remembering and forgetting: In what ways has Shaar Ha'aliya's past actively been transmitted to the present generation? Has it been accepted as meaningful? Or, conversely, has it been rejected, or even not conveyed? According to Yerushalmi, collective forgetting is when "human groups fail—whether purposely or passively, out of rebellion, indifference, or indolence, or as the result of some disruptive historical catastrophe—to transmit what they know out of the past to their posterity."[101] True, there is no memorialization at the site of Shaar Ha'aliya, but its story most certainly is being transmitted. In so many ways and through so many mediums, it is deeply embedded in Israeli historical remembrances. It is safe to say that among those doing the remembering, it has been accepted as meaningful. However, as of yet, it has not been accepted as meaningful by many others outside that circle and certainly not yet by the state itself.

Despite the richness of the remembrances, the abundant memorialization so close by, at Atlit, makes the Shaar Ha'aliya space seem practically barren. But Atlit also makes it clear just how challenging it would be
to include the memory of Shaar Ha'aliya in the Israeli landscape. This is
easy to grasp simply by imagining what a national heritage site at Shaar
Ha'aliya would look like if it were modeled on Atlit. The cabins and conditions would be practically identical, with rows of beds, lack of privacy,
and a general, material poverty of daily life. In fact, the conditions in the
Shaar Ha'aliya tents and cabins would be worse (dirtier, more ragged) than
Atlit. At Shaar Ha'aliya, there would be barbed wire. There wouldn't be an
actual watchtower, but there would be a gate and guards. But in this case,
the guards would be Israeli Jews. The Atlit remembrances emphasize the
Palmach raid on the camp in October 1945 and the liberation of the immigrants who were detained there. A heroic image of immigrants breaking
out of captivity could still be maintained in Shaar Ha'aliya by recreating
scenes of people crawling out under the barbed wire. In this way, the Shaar
Ha'aliya museum would keep the same image of the detained or isolated
Jews as either heroes or victims. But those images of the Jews behind barbed
wire in Atlit are complicated by the idea that if the people *inside* the
barbed wire are perceived as heroes and victims, then wouldn't that make
the people keeping them there oppressors? This is an easy image for Israel
when the guards are British but not when those guards are Israelis. And if
the barbed wire at Atlit is uncomplicated and easily reconcilable within the
Jewish Israeli story, the barbed wire at Shaar Ha'aliya is anything but. It is
fiercely complicated and dissonant.

The fact is that the themes that are such an inseparable part of how
Atlit is remembered are an equally inseparable part of how Shaar Ha'aliya
is remembered: Jews arriving in the land of / State of Israel should not
have been put behind barbed wire; the immigrants in the camp have been
treated poorly, and the people who put them there are to blame. Because
the architects of Atlit were British and the detainees were Jewish, these

memories reinforce existing Jewish Israeli national identity, which helps explain the elaborate heritage site. Yet the architects of Shaar Ha'aliya were Israeli and the detainees were Jewish Israelis. This dissonance helps explain the absence of a national heritage site. The criticism of Israel (that is an indelible part of those memories) and the image of the fence as a symbol of exclusion (that is an indelible part of that criticism) makes it clear how challenging it will be to integrate this history into the mainstream Israeli story.

Under Quarantine

It is hard to say whether Capa knew that what he had photographed was not just a solitary encounter, but certainly he knew that something meaningful was taking place. While the people and this fence are universal images of isolation, defiance, and humanity, they are also part of the particular story of Israel's establishment and its immigration experiment.

It is not difficult to understand those who stick to the framework of Israel's official international quarantine stations and leave Shaar Ha'aliya out of the equation. Yet this book has attempted to show how much we lose if we stay only within the confines of this limited definition and how much we gain by looking beyond it. This is where the story of Shaar Ha'aliya lies. Beyond is where assumptions about what defines a quarantine are challenged. Beyond is where we find questions about the persistence and evolution of this basic human act in the mid–twentieth century, during a period where practitioners of medical science largely believed that they were on the path to conquering infectious disease. By simply saying that Shaar Ha'aliya was not an official quarantine or that these lay-people were defining it wrong or that their references were only rhetoric and metaphor, we ignore the intricacies of this conflict. We ignore what it meant to the people as they were saying it, enforcing it, and defying it; what it meant to the society taking part in this discussion; and what it meant about the very concept of quarantine. As the story of Shaar Ha'aliya

illustrates, quarantine is not always as straightforward as a particular public health policy. It is an act of exclusion, a perceived "salvation for a threatened society," a "warding off," a barrier put in place to isolate both social
and biological contagion, and it is a cagey disciplinary mechanism that is
at once protective and punitive.[1]

The structure we see in the Capa photograph, the barbed wire fence
of the Shaar Ha'aliya quarantine, was built long before there was a Shaar
Ha'aliya. As the boundary for St. Luke's, it was a part of the intentionally inhospitable exterior of a military camp. When Palestine became
Israel and St. Luke's became Shaar Ha'aliya, that fence, which was kept in
place, took on a new dimension. It remained an intentionally inhospitable
exterior, but now it was part of a place that many people expected to be
uniquely hospitable.

The photograph gives us a glimpse of the conflicts that surrounded this
quarantine. The fence was there, it was meant to keep people out, but to
a large extent it simply did not. People went under it and through it; they
used it as a way to bypass the camp's official entrance and to come and
go as they pleased. Sylvia Meltzer described this act so simply: "I always
entered and exited through a hole in the fence." As such, it became a site
where power was negotiated. By keeping it intact, the state was asserting
authority while testing the limits of that authority. There would be a barrier, which was a real and intimidating presence, but they would not do
much more than that to prevent people like Sylvia from going through
it—there would be neither arrests nor fines. Through the act of breaking
in and out, the immigrants showed that not only did they belong in Israel
but Israel belonged to them: the various barriers, physical and otherwise,
really were in no position to keep them out. In trying to make the fence a
more serious obstacle, the police were working to assert their own power.
They were there to maintain order, but without certain measures in place
and functioning properly, such as a fence or a wall, they could not do their
job and, as far as they were concerned, they might as well not even be there.

It could be argued that the police and the state ultimately won this battle. By 1951, at least a partial wall was being built. At the end of that same year, selective immigration was implemented. This policy really did keep immigrants out of Israel. Nevertheless, the immigrants' persistent and ubiquitous protest at Shaar Ha'aliya must be seen in and of itself as victorious. Amnon Rubinstein has asserted that "protest is needed not as a means to immediate political action but as an almost symbolic rejection of deadlock."[2] Immigrant protest in Shaar Ha'aliya was bold, effective, and empowered. This is enough to make it significant.

Beyond the struggle over the physical structure was the struggle over meaning. Was the Shaar Ha'aliya quarantine a protective measure? Was it a normative act needed to guard the Yishuv against the real threat of dangerous contagious disease? Or was it punitive? Was it an unjustifiable act of isolation that threatened the inclusive ideal of the Jewish state? These were some of the issues that the fence led people to explore. The arguments were passionate, conflicted, and unresolved. That the immigrants arriving at this time were very sick is a point that is largely agreed upon by historians. In addition, it is also largely agreed that the absorbing society was uncomfortable about how the immigrants would influence the country. But if we step back for a moment, away from the atmosphere of near panic that clearly was prevalent, the actual epidemiological data leaves questions about how great a health risk these immigrants truly posed. Let's look again at a quote that we saw earlier: "Were Dr. Berman to know of the number of diseases that we are treating at Shaar Ha'aliya among the immigrants, and among them the number of contagious diseases, you would also think differently and you would say, along with us, that our government must close the camp in a thorough manner for the sake of the Yishuv and for the sake of the immigrants."[3] Although this particular quote is from Kalman Levin, he was not the only one making the argument. Given the medical treatment available and the medical infrastructure in place in Israel at the time, did trachoma, ringworm, tuberculosis, syphilis, head lice, and scabies (the most prevalent diseases at Shaar Ha'aliya) really justify such claims? Moreover, did this position make sense in light of the breaches in the fence by the thousands of people who were "under" the quarantine, like the man in Capa's photograph? The breaches make it clear that the protective argument was faulty, since the fence was not actually preventing contact between the immigrants and the rest of Israel.

These contradictions are well-suited to the history of quarantine, which raises problems about how illness is defined, who is doing the defining, as well as disparities between who is, and who is not, isolated. The contradictions are also well-suited to the history of post-1948 Israel, which was a time of dramatic change and instability. The chaotic environment that Shaar Ha'aliya became was a product of this period in Israel's history. As the Mapai workers described, conditions ranged "from difficult to very difficult," with overcrowding, disorderly and exhausting lines, uncomfortable conditions in the tents, and a surrounding barbed wire fence. Here was a young country that had just emerged from a cataclysmic war in grave financial straits, whose bureaucratic bodies and administration were just beginning to learn how to function, that was rapidly being transformed by an extraordinary number of immigrants from diverse backgrounds. To cope with these changes, the Israeli leadership looked to civic and medical policies that previously had been tested throughout the world, such as isolation as a part of immigration control. While it is relatively easy to sit back today and see that the health fears were likely exaggerated, there is no question that these fears were present in Israeli society at the time. From this perspective, quarantine was a salvation. It offered a powerful authority, a method of control and isolation that was fortified by its link to medical authority.

Yet in addition to the fear and instability, this was also a time of great idealism and excitement. For many people, the fact that a Jewish state actually existed and would now take in Jewish refugees—who most countries did not want—was awe-inspiring. From this perspective, the barbed wire fence was a demoralizing symbol of exclusion that repeatedly evoked comparisons with European DP camps and—worse—concentration camps. As such, the argument that quarantine was a protection was not convincing. To paraphrase Refael Sela, disease is not the only thing that is powerful and destructive—so is the symbolism of barbed wire, a fence, and a wall. It would seem that the different perspectives on this argument, like the Capa image, can be distilled down to fundamental and bold images: salvation, disease, imprisonment, oppression, liberation.

Shaar Ha'aliya has a place in contemporary Israeli culture. The historical remembrances that explore its story are varied and rich but largely bleak. Even Chava Alberstein's song, "Sharalia," one of the most popular and lighthearted representations of the camp, describes it as "a grey place with no color, no view." On the opposite end is the movie *The Ringworm Children*, which describes it as a type of prison where innocent children were subjected to coercive and traumatizing medical procedures. In this movie, we see the continued associations between Shaar Ha'aliya and a concentration camp, which was a recurring theme in the 1950s. Shaar Ha'aliya's depiction in these historical remembrances challenges persistent idealizations of Israeli history. Nowhere is this better understood than at the site of Atlit, that "harmonious model of the past," which is celebrated, so prominently, in the Israeli national space. The barbed wire at Atlit is memorialized in much the same way that the barbed wire fence at Shaar Ha'aliya is remembered: as unkind and repressive. In literature, memoirs, film, song, and personal testimonies, there is a recurring image of Shaar Ha'aliya as an isolated, demoralizing space, and there is persistent disappointment that Jews, finally arriving at the Jewish state, would be detained there. Mia Abramov described how, after "the relief of freedom," the amazing feeling of reaching the Jewish state, the thought of being put behind barbed wire at Shaar Ha'aliya was "incomprehensible." Considering how Shaar Ha'aliya is remembered and how Atlit has been memorialized, it is perhaps not surprising that Shaar Ha'aliya is currently neglected as a historic site. Robert Capa's photograph depicts a powerful image of people defying oppression that would easily fit into the narrative conveyed at the

Atlit Heritage Site, of Jews being subjected to, and then defying, British oppression. With such an uncomfortable story to tell, it is perhaps not surprising that the state prefers not to tell it and has let the historic site of Shaar Ha'aliya all but disappear. Nevertheless, we cannot fully understand Israel without understanding Shaar Ha'aliya. The largest, most concentrated space in which new Israelis encountered their new country, it was where this unusual nation of immigrants was first forged. It is at the heart of the Israeli story.

The Shaar Ha'aliya Memorial for Migrants and Medicine

I write these words in the midst of central Illinois. This is a quiet and lovely city, described by Tony Judt as an "oasis,"[1] with miles and miles of cornfields lying between this town and any major metropolis. What with snow, cornfields, and quiet, my home in Israel feels very far away.

Even from this distance, when I stop and take a moment to consider the politics that would play a part in a Shaar Ha'aliya museum, it's enough to make my head hurt. This story brings to the surface some of contemporary Israel's most unsettled social, ethnic, and political conflicts: racism toward immigrants from Muslim and Arab countries, hostility toward Holocaust survivors, the trauma of ringworm treatment, and through the question of walls between peoples, the separation barrier between Israel and Palestine. There is not a doubt in my mind that discussions about Shaar Ha'aliya today would be just as divisive as they were in the 1950s. But I am far, and it is quiet, so I'll allow myself to daydream.

The memorial I envision would not be like Atlit. It would not be grandiose or expensive. In my mind, it would be mostly photographs, large, outdoors, that would capture people's interest and entice them to stop for a moment as they passed by. There would be quotes from the immigrants and workers that convey, so poignantly and so honestly, what this place was like. It would include photographs of the moving encounters at the Haifa port, with people beaming as they finally reached Israel and with

others hugging loved ones who had been waiting. There would be photographs of life in the camp itself, of young people smiling, stretched out
in the sun; of an elegant man in sunglasses, walking arm in arm with a
woman while holding a musical instrument wrapped in a burlap sack. But
there would also be photographs of hundreds of people waiting in grueling lines; of children—bald, miserable looking—being treated for ringworm; of crowded, dirty cabins; and of the barbed wire fence, tall and
unwelcoming, with people crawling under.[2]

It would be called the Shaar Ha'aliya Memorial for Migrants and Medicine,[3] and one of its aims would be to use the particular story of Shaar
Ha'aliya as a way to stimulate conversation about contemporary stories
of the medically defended exclusion of outsiders. This would be done
through quotes and photographs that highlight parallels between the two.
For example, in 1951, to defend the quarantine of immigrants at Shaar
Ha'aliya, Pinchas Yorman said this: "Now, let's imagine to ourselves that
Shaar Ha'aliya were wide open and anyone and everyone would come
and go [. . .] This would mean that an immigrant with active tuberculosis would ride on a busy public bus to Haifa and to any other place. The
same with eye diseases, sexually transmitted diseases, etc."[4] In 2009, to
defend the deportation of Israeli-born children of migrant workers, Eli
Yishai, then Israel's interior minister, said this: "Hundreds of thousands of
foreign workers will come here now . . . with hepatitis, tuberculosis, mea-
sles, AIDS [. . .] Doesn't that threaten the Zionist project of the State of
Israel?"[5] In both these cases, we see "foreigners" threatening Israeli society
with their "dangerous diseases." In 2009, the menacing presence was the
children of migrant workers, who are "threatening" because they are not
Jewish. In 1951, the menacing presence was Israel's new immigrants (Holocaust survivors and immigrants from Arab and Muslim countries), who
were threatening because they did not fit into the image of healthy, strong,
European Zionists. The privilege of hindsight helps us put the story from
the 1950s in perspective as a fear that may have had roots in logic and the
context of the time, but that was in fact irrational and disproportionate to

the perceived risk. As I pointed out in a 2009 op-ed piece, this hindsight allows us to see more clearly the problems with Yishai's later comments:

> Yishai's current use of this rhetoric is both ironic and alarming. The irony is that a person who is proud and vocal about his 'Mizrahi' heritage would resort to the same discriminatory, inflammatory rhetoric that was so painfully used against 'Mizrahim' in the past, including—in all likelihood—Yishai's own family. The alarm is that coming from the interior minister, this rhetoric is no longer just inflammatory but also dangerous; it instills irrational fear in the minds of the public and encourages further discrimination against an already socially marginalized group.
>
> Much wisdom is to be gained from historical knowledge. In this case, we have seen that a child whose "diseases" threaten the State of Israel can overcome this irrational stigma to obtain great achievements. Just imagine—he can even become interior minister.[6]

The historical perspective of a memorial for migrants and medicine would offer a way to reconsider the fears from our own time, which might seem so logical to us. It would force a discussion on the particular impact of these types of claims, such as those made by Kalman Levin and Eli Yishai, which link disease and foreignness as a great threat and, as such, take power from biomedicine as a justification for exclusion.

Like so many other countries, Israel needs a space for this type of reflection. It needs to publically confront incidents where blood donations by immigrants from Ethiopia were discarded by the Magen David Adom (Israel's Red Cross) because of a policy that singled them out as a high-risk group for AIDS;[7] where, more recently, other immigrants from Ethiopia were given injections of the long acting contraceptive Depo-Provera without informed consent;[8] of the ringworm story, which still continues to resonate; and of the children of migrant workers who the interior minister publically and irrationally demonized as an ominous public health threat. Israelis need to see these acts as part of larger trends of exclusion. We need to step out from behind the frightening frame of disease and the authoritative shield of medicine to confront the contemporary stereotypes and prejudices that allow for these acts of isolation and discrimination. There would also be room to explore important successes, such as the groundbreaking Ringworm Victims' Compensation Law from 1994, which established that people who were treated for ringworm in the 1950s are entitled to monetary restitution from the state.[9] Including the ringworm law would show a direct thread between the history of disease and medicine at Shaar Ha'aliya and later acknowledgment of the medical shortcomings and regrets for how this history played out.

Howard Markel has written about "the persistent association between immigrants and disease in American society."[10] The Shaar Ha'aliya memorial would offer an opportunity to consider this idea in Israeli society, as well as part of a global phenomenon: simply the persistent association between immigrants and disease in society. The memorial that I envision would show both the universal and particular angles to these stories. It could bring in stories from other societies where migrants and minorities have been targeted as carriers of dangerous contagion: Chinese and Southeast Asian Canadian communities and SARS; gays and Haitians and AIDS in the United States; West Africans and Ebola.

This memorial would also have to include a broader discussion of isolation and otherness, beyond the confines of medicine and health, since the idea of a barrier in Israel is more relevant than ever. It seems to me almost impossible to read Refael Sela's words from 1951 without considering them in context with contemporary discussions about Israel's wall with Palestine: "The wall is a symbol that no explanation can negate: a symbol of division between peoples."[11]

These are not easy issues to confront. I am sure that some people will be deeply troubled by the thought of linking them together, but I would love for this memorial to rise to the challenge. I would love for it to be a place where Israeli-born children of Ethiopian immigrants, migrant workers from the Philippines, Sudanese refugees in Holot, internally displaced Palestinian-Israelis and immigrants from Russia can find their own stories reflected—where they can find some sort of identification and see something of their own experiences celebrated, alongside those of immi-grants from Morocco, Romania, Iraq, Egypt, and Poland, whose families actually went through the camp. I would love for the people who can't iden-tify with Atlit's pioneers to drive a few miles north and find themselves in the pictures of Shaar Ha'aliya's migrants.

I have no illusions that this place will miraculously fix Israel's problems, that people will come away from this memorial holding hands, seeing the error of their ways, and embracing one another's differences. In fact, while writing this book, I have struggled with the issue of noncommemoration at the site of Shaar Ha'aliya. I've wondered whether I'm exaggerating the importance of a museum. Perhaps the rich remembrances that are a part of the Israeli social and cultural landscapes are enough? But I am not con-vinced. The more I spend time with this issue, the more strongly I believe that, as long as so much space and energy is devoted to centers like Atlit and the Yad Vashem Holocaust museum, the absence of a national site to embrace Shaar Ha'aliya is shameful. It is worth considering: If the immi-grants at Shaar Ha'aliya had been resisting the Turks, the British, Germans, or Arabs, wouldn't this history have been glorified a long time ago?[12]

David Biale has written of historical criticism that it "can liberate us from the burden of a mythical past, while at the same time presenting us with a new past that we may have not considered."[13]

The stories of Shaar Ha'aliya's immigrants are stories of strong, vul-nerable, and simple humanity: a mother climbing into a locked clinic to steal away her son and nurse him back to health in Shaar Ha'aliya's meager tents and TB patients staging a hunger strike. They offer a rich, compli-cated new past that is certainly worth considering.

Of course, I keep coming back to Capa's photograph of the man crawl-ing under the barbed wire fence, but another photograph also comes to mind, of an adult man washing up. This man is sitting on a stool, next to a large sink, as another man tends to his hair, maybe cutting it. Both are dressed in long trousers. The man sitting has a smock over his clothes to protect them as his hair is being done, while the man standing is

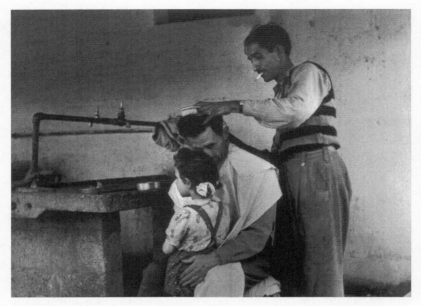

Figure 9. An intimate moment inside the camp. © Robert Capa/Magnum Photos.

wearing a sweater-vest over a button down shirt. Their cared-for appearance contrasts with the cement, mud, and filth in the washing room. The seated man has his arm around a small girl who is wearing a ribbon in her hair. This gesture is protective and comforting. The gentleness of the embrace, the intimacy of people helping to groom one another, the ribbon in the girl's hair, the fabric covering the man's clothes all come together to create a touching portrait of people trying to maintain human refinement and dignity in Shaar Ha'aliya's unrefined conditions. These acts of heroism need to be celebrated.

Acknowledgments

I was introduced to the field of medical history through the research of my father, William Edward Seidelman. In our home in Hamilton, where my father was a professor of family medicine at McMaster University, I grew up seeing, firsthand, how meaningful and exciting this discipline could be. Indeed, there is no scholar whose work has had a greater influence on my own work than my father. I have loved and benefited from decades of reading his articles, listening to his lectures, and having conversations with him. Although the subject matter and region of my scholarship are different from his, I hope that when he sees commitment and excitement coming through in my book he recognizes his own imprint.

There is no person who has had a greater impact on me and my intellectual and personal achievements than my beautiful mother, Racheline Dayan Seidelman. I am so fortunate to have had her conversation, wisdom, love, advocacy, and sass to rely on throughout my life. When I think of the immigrants at Shaar Ha'aliya, I think of my mother's own immigration story, the difficult changes that were forced upon her and her extraordinary resilience. And although everyone in my family is an avid reader, my mother's relationship with books is the one that I most admire. I have learned from her to read broadly, to read critically, and to savor books. I am glad to be giving her an additional book to savor.

Everything I am and everything I have accomplished is because of my parents. They showed me and my sisters the value of intellectual and creative pursuits and then they gave us their support when we followed these pursuits on various unusual paths. They gave us a home filled with love, warmth, respect, stimulation, debate, integrity, and fun. Even as I am distanced from this home by years and oceans, I always carry it with me.

———

This project developed out of my PhD at Ben-Gurion University of the Negev; I wrote this under the guidance of my advisors, Shifra Shvarts and S. Ilan Troen. I have learned so much from them—more than I can fully express—and I am grateful for all that they have done to help me.

I went through the PhD at Ben-Gurion University together with my dear friends Nimrod Zinger and Ari Barell. I am better off for their years of friendship, excellent advice, and enriching dialogue. Similarly, Nadav Davidovitch has been a generous friend and teacher to me from the days of our shared office overlooking the Negev desert. Early on in my PhD, it was my good fortune to be introduced to Allan M. Brandt when he spent a few weeks at Ben-Gurion University as a visiting distinguished professor. Allan's compassion never ceases to amaze me. I am incredibly grateful to him for his kind words and magnanimous expressions of support. I would not be where I am today without his years of mentorship.

Toward the end of my time at BGU, I was fortunate to work as a research assistant to David Ohana and Michael Feige z"l. I cherish those days spent at the Sde Boker campus. My time was divided working serenely under the portrait of Ben-Gurion in the library and snatching breaks outside to take in the Zin Valley's extraordinary vista. When I needed a diversion from all the quiet, I would visit David's office as he and Michael shared impassioned (and not at all quiet) exchanges on Israeli history. I learned so much from them about Israel, writing books, and the joys of work and friendship.

But these fond memories are laced with terrible sadness: Michael Feige—a gentle man of peace and humanism—was killed in a terrorist attack in Tel Aviv in 2016. I will always see Michael as a role model for what scholars of Israel should be and how teachers should conduct themselves. I can't say that I am always successful at implementing the lessons I learned from Michael. But I have them in my mind as examples to try to live up to. One of the last interactions I had with Michael Feige was at a conference in California when he took me aside to kindly ask about the progress I was making on this book. I wish I could have finished it in time for him to read it, but I am profoundly grateful that I had the opportunity to work with and learn from this special man.

I began the process of turning my dissertation into a book while I was teaching at the University of Illinois at Urbana-Champaign. I could not have hoped for a more supportive and stimulating environment than the Program for Jewish Culture and Society. I always looked forward to the monthly workshops, where I gained an immeasurable amount from the rigorous and lively intellectual exchanges. Over the years, Gene Avrutin, Harriet Murav, Bruce Rosenstock, and Brett Kaplan warmly and repeatedly shared guidance and friendship. Michael Rothberg, Virginia Dominguez, Dara E. Goldman, Jonathan Druker, Zia Miric, Ofira Fuchs, and Jordan Finkin were kind colleagues who I always enjoyed encountering and whose insight during the workshops pushed me to think in different directions. Similarly, my wonderful colleagues in history, Craig Koslofsky, Peter Fritzsche, and Leslie Reagan, shared generous advice and illuminating conversations.

I am grateful to the numerous people at the University of Illinois who took time to read and comment on drafts of chapters that I presented in the history workshop and the Program for Jewish Culture and Society. I was also fortunate to take part in the First Book Writing Group led by the late Nancy Abelmann and Craig Koslofsky. Independent of any workshop, Craig Koslofsky and Dana Rabin generously commented on an early draft of chapter 4. Peter Fritzsche and Gene Avrutin went above and beyond by reading and responding to the entire manuscript. I am incredibly grateful to them for their suggestions and encouragement. Thank you to Lee Melhado for diligently proofreading an early version of my manuscript and for heroically trying, against all odds, to teach me how to use a semicolon.

I am particularly glad to finally be able to publically express my gratitude to Dana Rabin and Matti Bunzl. Dana's friendship and mentorship have been vital sources of support to me as I wrote this book. And without Matti Bunzl, all of these important experiences for me in Illinois would never have happened. From the earliest emails we exchanged, he exuded an enthusiasm and warm welcome. In his then capacity as director of the Program of Jewish Culture and Society, he immediately made me feel a part of the program, and he took time to help introduce me to the culture of academia in the United States, which was foreign to me. He was excited about my book project, and he helped me find my way through it. The word I recall Matti saying often is "fabulous." It suits him.

———

The University of Oklahoma has been such a surprising and wonderful home to me since I had the good fortune to move here in 2015. I work alongside colleagues whose scholarship and priorities I admire and whose company I enjoy, and I teach students who are bright, intellectually curious, and hardworking. I want to thank the Schusterman family for their commitment to the Schusterman Center in Judaic and Israel Studies and, specifically, for endowing the chair that I now hold. Thank you to our provost, Kyle Harper, for sharing thoughts on the history of disease—which I benefited from and very much enjoyed. Thank you to our dean, David Wrobel, and our associate dean, Vicki Sturtevant, for their exceptional kindness and support. And thank you to my many students who, with their good cheer, have helped introduce me to the fascinating facets of Oklahoma life.

My history chair, James S. Hart, is one of a kind. His kindness and encouragement during difficult periods of this writing process were a special expression of *menschkeit*. Alan Levenson, the director of the Schusterman Center, has been a welcoming and generous colleague. While I regret that my time here did not overlap more with Noam Stillman's, I have fond memories of the way he and Dina warmly received me and my family when we first arrived. Thank you to David Chappelle for being such a wonderful friend, sharing time and indulgent discussions, and then closely reading my manuscript at a time when I most needed his feedback. Alan Levenson and Rafie Folsom's comments on different sections of my manuscript were similarly valuable and deeply appreciated. A special thank you to my fantastic departmental mentor Sandie Holguin for her excellent, supportive, and fun advice. I am so fortunate that Jennifer Davis's door was always open at the times I most needed her sage and incisive guidance and her uplifting laughter. Even if her office was hidden behind long corridors in a dusty attic, I would still seek her out. Janie Adkins, Christa Seedorf, and Tryce Hyman do such a fantastic job of running the history department and the Judaic Studies center that I would be lost without them. No less important, they make the office a place that I look forward to going to. To all the members of Committee G, I am so grateful for your camaraderie, intelligence, and fabulousness. Indeed I want to thank all my wonderful colleagues in history at the University of Oklahoma. Your guidance, friendship, and advice have helped me bring this project to a happy close.

It has been a sincere pleasure to work with Elisabeth Maselli at Rutgers University Press. Her support has been crucial in getting this book published. I deeply appreciate her exceptional professionalism, her excitement about my work, and her great kindness. Thank you to Jennifer Shaiman and Helen Walsh for their expert assistance in preparing the manuscript for production. And thank you to the Office of the Vice President for Research, The University of Oklahoma, for providing funding to support this publication.

The friendship of many people who I love and admire sustained me while writing this book, as it has throughout my life. Beth Hill, Rae Bates, and Ruthie Spinner are my roots from Hamilton. Simona Di Nepi and Miriam Orelle were students with me at the Hebrew University. I am so fortunate to still have them all to turn to and laugh with after so many decades. Simon Lichman, Rivanna Miller, and their whole crew profoundly shaped my perspective on Israel (and humanity) while sharing wonderful conversations and cups of tea. Laura Sola, Wendy Mathewson, and Jenna Zieman made life on Urbana's California Avenue a magical time. Bridget Love and Sam Temple cushioned our bumpy arrival in Oklahoma with love and pastries (the same thing?). And Becca Waggoner and Myongjin Kim have recently come into my life as I adjust with my family to a happy, settled state in Norman.

My greatest debt is to my families—the Seidelmans and Pincus. My two fabulous sisters, Aviva Dayan and Ayela Seidelman are my role models, sparring partners, and cherished friends. They believed in me and encouraged me through the many years of writing this book. I am so lucky to have them in my life. Their husbands, Ehav Ever and Bari Moscovitz, have added new and wonderful dimensions to our family. (I am especially glad that Bari is now old enough to read this book. It feels like only yesterday that he was a young toddler). Libi, Ellie, Ofri, Elinour, and Renana—my magnificent nieces and nephew have expanded our family in the most wonderful ways. I love you very much.

At some point in my PhD, I was welcomed into the Pincu family. Yehuda, Dalia, Yossi, Yaron, Nir—and later, lovely Chen and my beloved nephews Maor and Beeri—took me in with their boundless love. After long days in the library, Shabbat dinners at the Pincu home—raucous, delicious, and overflowing with laughter—were a restorative distraction. My wonderful parents-in-law, Yehuda and Dalia, have been a particular source of support. They flew across oceans to give love and care to infants, children, and exhausted new parents as Yair and I struggled with the challenges of parenthood and careers. Yehuda and Dalia watched me write from a careful distance and—with their infinite generosity—always made it clear that they are proud of me. I am so grateful to them.

Most important are the great loves of my life. My dazzling children, Shalev and Gefen, fill my world with abundant joy. I absolutely adore you. And finally, Yair Pincu. Everything about life is better with him in it. When writing this book was hard, he helped push me through. When writing this book was wonderful, he shared my joy. There was not a single moment that he didn't have my back. I know this and felt this, and I am inordinately grateful.

Notes

INTRODUCTION

1. *Oxford English Dictionary*, 1st ed. (1961), s.v. "quarantine" (my emphasis).

2. Moshe Lissak, *The Mass Immigration in the Fifties: The Failure of the Melting Pot Policy* [in Hebrew] (Jerusalem: Bialik Institute, 1999), 26; Dvora Hacohen, *Immigrants in Turmoil: The Great Wave of Immigration to Israel and Its Absorption, 1948–1953* [in Hebrew] (Jerusalem: Yad Yitzhak Ben Tzvi, 1994), 82; Shifra Shvarts, *Kupat-Holim, the Histadrut and the Government* [in Hebrew] (Sde Boker, Israel: Ben-Gurion Research Center, 2000), 163. In *A Home for All Jews*, Orit Rozin refers to it as a camp "where immigrants were received and sorted" (Orit Rozin, *A Home for All Jews: Citizenship, Rights, and National Identity in the New Israeli State* [Waltham, Mass.: Brandeis University Press, 2016], 123).

3. The first was an anonymous reader's comment on my dissertation, and the second was an anonymous reviewer's comment to an early draft of what became my article, "Conflicts of Quarantine: The Case of Jewish Immigrants to the Jewish State," *American Journal of Public Health* 102, no. 2 (2012): 243–252.

4. Alan M. Kraut, *Silent Travellers: Germs, Genes and the Immigrant Menace* (Baltimore: Johns Hopkins University Press, 1994).

5. *Yishuv* is the term used to refer to the Jewish community in Palestine prior to the establishment of the state of Israel. Its use also appears in reference to the Jewish community in Israel in the state's early years.

6. Though the question of regulating the scope and makeup of the immigration was being discussed both by policy makers and the public as early as the fall of 1948, during the initial years of statehood, a definitive selection policy was not implemented. Dvora Hacohen explains that decisions by the Jewish Agency to

regulate immigration came in early 1949. Avi Picard has documented how, following years of discussion and debate, a selective immigration policy was finally implemented in November 1951. Picard clarifies that this policy was considered a temporary arrangement until the state could be stabilized, and Hacohen emphasizes that this policy was always conditional to there being no danger to the Jews in their country of origin. If Jews were endangered in the countries they were living in, the selection policy was invalid. Thus the debate came down to determining whether a community was indeed in danger and in need of being rescued. Avi Picard, Yishay Arnon, and Haim Malka have shown that the repercussions of these decisions were occasionally disastrous, particularly in the case of Morocco and communist Europe. But even as the regulation policy kept many people out, and the rate of immigration plateaued, the numbers of immigrants continued to be substantial. Moshe Lissak's figures show that in the years 1952–1956, more than eighty thousand immigrants moved to Israel.

7. As is widely discussed, the first scholars to study the mass immigration were Israeli sociologists. Dvora Hacohen's early work *Immigrants in Turmoil* was a watershed moment where historians of Israel began to see the mass immigration as a topic worthy of careful historical reflection and the post-1948 immigrants themselves as important agents within the Israeli landscape whose particular experiences needed to be understood through archival research. Of course, it also makes sense that historical studies did not begin until this point because enough time had to pass to allow for historical reflection and the opening of archives. Some of the important scholars whose historical studies followed closely after, or were contemporaneous to Hacohen, are Tzvi Tzameret, Yaron Tzur, Mordechai Naor, and Dalia Ofer.

8. Avi Picard's illuminating *Cut to Measure* focuses on North African immigrants, particularly those from Morocco and Tunisia. Esther Meir and, more recently, Orit Bashkin have written invaluable studies on the experiences of immigrants from Iraq; in his study of Argentinian immigration, Sebastian Klor shows the value of looking at the immigrants who arrived to Israel in smaller numbers; Hanna Yablonka's groundbreaking work came earlier. Yablonka's focus has been on the integration of Holocaust survivors in Israeli society; the anthology of works by Egyptian-Israeli author Jacqueline Kahanoff adds to our understanding of the immigration of Egyptian Jews to Israel.

9. Shifra Shvarts is the preeminent scholar on the history of medicine in Israel. Her numerous studies have fundamentally changed the way we understand the Israeli health care system. Sachlav Stoler-Liss continued in Shvarts' path, with her important scholarship on health promotion and health education during the

mass immigration. Nadav Davidovitch has become a unique and commanding voice in this field, consistently and persuasively questioning systems of power and medical hegemony. Rakefet Zalashik has written the preeminent study on the history of psychiatry in Israel. Historian Ari Barell's important study on the role of science and technology in Israeli nation-building has led to his fascinating new research on Israel's Iron Dome antirocket technology. Nurit Kirsch's important work on genetics straddles both the history of medicine and the history of science. Orit Rozin's work has introduced the social historian's discipline to the study of mass immigration. Anat Helman's study of everyday life in 1950s Israel offers an exciting new take on the culture into which the new immigrants arrived.

10. Two recent publications that do an exemplary job overcoming a simplistic Ashkenazi/Mizrahi discourse are Orit Bashkin's *Impossible Exodus* and Avi Picard's *Cut to Measure*. Picard unearthed sources that carefully document the details surrounding Israel's selective immigration policy from the end of 1951—a policy that had disastrous repercussions for immigrants from North Africa. He places them within a broad historical context that defies any possibilities for a reductive perception of the Mizrahi or Ashkenazi experience. The result is an illuminating and erudite historiography. Bashkin has made the immigrant's own experience central to her research. One of the many important contributions of this exceptional book are the sections where the author examines the creation of the Mizrahi identity, asking what exactly this identity is and how it developed within the Israeli experience for post-1948 immigrants.

11. Orit Bashkin, *Impossible Exodus: Iraqi Jews in Israel* (Stanford: Stanford University Press, 2017), 13. This approach of breaking the larger frame of Mizrahi and, similarly, Ashkenazi to examine the particular experiences of distinct immigrant groups could provide a useful entry for additional inquiries into Shaar Ha'aliya.

12. Ibid., 182.

13. Ibid., 212.

14. "Mizrahi solidarity in Israel was forged in the transit camps, schools, kibbutzim, and the Israeli labor market, and grew stronger through the protesting of the state's policies" (ibid., 209).

15. For example, immigrant camps, labor camps, and transit camps, or *ma'abarot*. See Lissak, *Mass Immigration in the Fifties*; Rozin, *A Home for All Jews*; Hacohen, *Immigrants in Turmoil*.

16. Central Zionist Archives (CZA), AK 456/3, "Account of Entry into Shaar Ha'aliya," 1955.

IMMIGRANTS TO ISRAEL AND SHAAR HA'ALIYA, 1948–1957

Year	Israel	Shaar Ha'aliya
1948	101,819	n/a
1949	239,076	97,840
1950	169,405	127,854
1951	173, 901	99,602
1952	23,375	14,342
1953	10,317	6,692
1954	17,471	5,338
1955	36,758	576
1956	55,494	No numbers available
1957	69,611	No numbers available

Sources: Numbers of immigrants to Israel: Jehuda Wallach and Moshe Lissak, eds., *Carta's Atlas of Israel: The First Years, 1948–1961* [in Hebrew] (Jerusalem: Carta and the Israeli Ministry of Defense, 1978), 73; numbers of immigrants to Shaar Ha'aliya: CZA, AK 456/3, "Account of Entry into Shaar Ha'aliya," 1955.

17. Reports from the World Health Organization (WHO) epidemiological radio bulletin transmissions were received at the Lod air terminal and transmitted to the quarantine stations. Theodor Grushka, *Health Services in Israel* (Jerusalem: Ministry of Health, 1968), 110.

18. Dan Bar-El, "Cholera Epidemics in Palestine, 1865–1918" [in Hebrew] (PhD diss., Bar-Ilan University, 2006); Dan Bar-El, *Ruah ra'ah: Magefot ha-kholerah ve-hitpathut ha-refu'ah be-Eretz-Yisrael beshalhei ha-tkufah ha-otmanit* [An ill wind: Cholera epidemics and medical development in Palestine in the late Ottoman period] (Jerusalem: Bialik Institute, 2010).

19. Nissim Levy, *The History of Medicine in the Holy Land: 1799–1948* [in Hebrew] (Israel: Hakibbutz Hameuhad, 1998), 515.

20. Grushka, *Health Services in Israel*, 110. "Body lice, which were occasionally found on immigrants during the period of mass immigration . . . have not been reported in recent years" (39).

21. Ibid., 39.

22. Michael A. Davies, "Health and Disease in Israel, 1948–1994," in *Health and Disease in the Holy Land: Studies in the History and Sociology of Medicine from Ancient Times to the Present*, ed. Manfred Waserman and Samuel S. Kottek (Lewiston, N.Y.:

Edwin Mellen, 1996), 443. Grushka writes that quarantinable diseases were "not endemic in Israel, and the usual internationally accepted procedures are adopted to prevent their introduction" (Grushka, *Health Services in Israel*, 39).

23. Grushka, *Health Services in Israel*, 109.

24. Levy, *History of Medicine*, 515.

25. Michel Foucault, *Discipline and Punish: The Birth of the Prison* (New York: Vintage Books, 1995).

26. "Cutting across modernity's pluralities, however, are three key characteristics of enforced isolation in the modern era: the flexibility of rationales for segregation or confinement, which often move seamlessly between punishment, protection and prevention; the careful consideration of isolation's architectural and spatial dimensions; and the subjectification of the isolated, both the official project of modern exclusion and a crucible for the cultivation of selfhood" (Carolyn Strange and Alison Bashford, eds., *Isolation: Places and Practices of Exclusion* [London: Routledge, 2003], 2).

27. Frédéric Charbonneau, "Quarantine and Caress," in *Imagining Contagion in Early Modern Europe*, ed. Claire L. Carlin (Basingstoke, U.K.: Palgrave Macmillan, 2005).

28. David F. Musto, "Quarantine and the Problem of AIDS," *Milbank Quarterly* 64, supp. 1 (1986): 98.

29. Ibid.

CHAPTER 1 — CONFINES

1. Central Zionist Archives (CZA), AK 456/3, Administrative Report #37, 28.9.51.

2. For population numbers for Palestine and Israel from 1517 to 2004, see Itamar Rabinovich and Jehuda Reinharz, eds., *Israel in the Middle East: Documents and Readings on Society, Politics and Foreign Relations, Pre-1948 to the Present*, 2nd ed. (Waltham, Mass.: Brandeis University Press, 2008), 571. On the 1948 war and the Palestinian refugees, see Benny Morris, *Righteous Victims: A History of the Zionist-Arab Conflict 1881–2001* (New York: Vintage Books, 2001); Benny Morris, *The Birth of the Palestinian Refugee Problem Revisited* (Cambridge: Cambridge University Press, 2004); Benny Morris, *1948 and After: Israel and the Palestinians* (New York: Oxford University Press, 1994). On Palestinian citizens of Israel, see Shira Robinson, *Citizen Strangers: Palestinians and the Birth of Israel's Liberal Settler State* (Stanford: Stanford University Press, 2013).

3. For the article that announced the beginning of the "New Historians," their revisions of contemporary understanding of the 1948 war, and an outline of the

major myths that shaped Jewish Israeli historiography, see Benny Morris, "The New Historiography: Israel Confronts Its Past," *Tikkun* 3, no 6 (1988): 19–23, 98–103.

4. For numbers on the mass immigration, see Jehuda Wallach and Moshe Lissak, eds., *Carta's Atlas of Israel: The First Years, 1948–1961* [in Hebrew] (Jerusalem: Carta and the Israeli Ministry of Defense, 1978), 73; Moshe Lissak, *The Mass Immigration in the Fifties: The Failure of the Melting Pot Policy* [in Hebrew] (Jerusalem: Bialik Institute, 1999), 3–4; *Encyclopedia Judaica*, 2nd ed., s.vv. "Aliyah and Absorption," "Immigration to Israel, 1948–1970"; Dvora Hacohen, *Immigrants in Turmoil: The Great Wave of Immigration to Israel and Its Absorption, 1948–1953* [in Hebrew] (Jerusalem: Yad Yitzhak Ben Tzvi, 1994), 323–328.

5. Hacohen, *Immigrants in Turmoil*, 323–324.

6. Israel's establishment occurred at a time in history that had left thousands of Jews needing refuge, with the dismantling of the displaced persons (DP) camps in Europe, the rise of Arab nationalism, the contraction of European colonial power, and the escalation of the Israeli-Arab conflict throughout the Middle East. (On the deterioration of life for Jews in Arab lands, see Hacohen, *Immigrants in Turmoil*, 3. On the rise of Arab nationalism and contraction of European colonial power on a global scale, see David Thompson, *Europe since Napoleon* [London: Penguin Books, 1990], 866–875; Todd Shepherd, *The Invention of Decolonization: The Algerian War and the Remaking of France* [Ithaca, N.Y.: Cornell University Press, 2006]). All these factors, taking place in the backdrop of the exhilaration and expectation among world Jewry surrounding the establishment of a Jewish state, played a part in the massive influx of Jewish immigrants to Israel following 1948. See Dvora Hacohen, "Mediniyut ha-aliyah ba-asor ha-rishon la-medinah: Ha-nisyonot le-hagbalat ha-aliyah ve-goralam" [Immigration policy in the first decade of statehood: The attempts to restrict immigration and their outcome], in *Kibbutz galuyot: Ha-aliyah le-Eretz Yisrael, mitos u-metzi'ut* [Ingathering of exiles: Aliyah to the Land of Israel, myth and reality], ed. Dvora Hacohen (Jerusalem: Zalman Shazar Center for Jewish History, 1998), 291.

7. Dvora Hacohen, "From Fantasy to Reality—Ben-Gurion's Plan for Mass Immigration, 1942–1945," *Research Institute for the History of the Keren Kayemeth LeIsrael* [Jewish National Fund Land and Settlement] 18 (October 1995).

8. Ibid., 5.

9. Ibid., 4.

10. Ibid.

11. Barry Rubin, *Israel: An Introduction* (New Haven, Conn.: Yale University Press, 2012), 25.

12. Defining the terms *native* and *immigrant* is a challenge when used in the context of Israeli Jews, particularly in this period. Dalia Ofer addresses the subjectivity

of this concept where people who had arrived in 1946–1947 were considered "veterans," whereas those who came after 1948 were "immigrants" (Dalia Ofer, ed., *Israel in the Great Wave of Immigration, 1948–1953* [in Hebrew] [Jerusalem: Yad Yitzhak Ben Tzvi, 1996]).

13. Hacohen, "Mediniyut ha-aliyah ba-asor ha-rishon la-medinah," 285. This ideal was expressed in the 1950 law of return: "Every Jew has the right to come to this country as an *oleh*." The text of the law of return can be found at http://www.jewishvirtuallibrary.org.

14. Irwin Shaw and Robert Capa, *Report on Israel* (New York: Simon & Schuster, 1950), 33.

15. For some accounts of the Altalena affair, see Morris, *Righteous Victims*, 236–237; Anita Shapira, ed., *We Hereby Declare: 60 Chosen Speeches in the History of Israel* [in Hebrew] (Or Yehuda, Israel: Kinneret, Zmora-Bitan, Dvir, 2008), 46–57; Jerold S. Auerbach, *Brothers at War: Israel and the Tragedy of the Altalena* (New Orleans: Quid Pro Books, 2011).

16. See "'Who Is a Jew?'—Professor Isaiah Berlin's Memorandum to the Prime Minister of Israel, 23 January 1959," *Israel Studies* 13, no. 3 (2008): 170–177; Howard Sachar, *A History of Israel from the Rise of Zionism to Our Time*, 3rd ed. (New York: Knopf, 2007), 602–608.

17. See Shira Robinson, *Citizen Strangers: Palestinians and the Birth of Israel's Liberal Settler State* (Stanford: Stanford University Press, 2013).

18. John Efron, Steven Weitzman, and Matthias Lehmann, *The Jews: A History*, 2nd ed. (New York: Routledge, 2016), 406.

19. For the political, social, economic, and military dimensions involved in Israel's establishment, see S. Ilan Troen and Noah Lucas, *Israel: The First Decade of Independence* (Albany: State University of New York Press, 1995). For the history of Israeli society during the mass immigration, see Orit Rozin, *The Rise of the Individual in 1950s Israel: A Challenge to Collectivism* (Waltham, Mass.: Brandeis University Press, 2011). On the shortage of health care workers and hospital beds, see Shifra Shvarts, *Health and Zionism: The Israeli Health Care System, 1948–1960* (Rochester, N.Y.: University of Rochester Press, 2008).

20. Anat Helman, *Becoming Israeli: National Ideals and Everyday Life in the 1950s* (Waltham, Mass.: Brandeis University Press, 2014), 47.

21. Ibid., 48.

22. Rozin, *Rise of the Individual*. For an earlier discussion of the austerity policy, see Nachum Gross, "Israel's Economy" [in Hebrew], in *The First Decade*, ed. Zvi Zameret and Hana Yablonka (Jerusalem: Yad Yitzhak Ben-Tzvi, 1997).

23. See "The Humorous Side of Rationing," in Helman, *Becoming Israeli*, 47–67; and "Human Material," in Orit Bashkin, *Impossible Exodus: Iraqi Jews in Israel*

(Stanford: Stanford University Press, 2017). Helman focuses on humor in the *Yishuv* and Bashkin focuses on humor found among Iraqi immigrants in the transit camps. Bashkin describes this as the immigrants using "one of the oldest mechanisms in the Jewish historical arsenal for dealing with difficult and absurd situations: their sense of humor" (Bashkin, *Impossible Exodus*, 30).

24. Lissak, *Mass Immigration*, 21.

25. Ibid., 26.

26. Moshe Sikron, "The Mass Immigration—Its Size, Characteristics and Influences," in *Immigrants and Transit Camps, 1948–1952*, ed. Mordechai Naor (Jerusalem: Yad Yitzhak Ben Zvi, 1986), 46.

27. Mordechai Naor explains that there were four types of transit camps (*ma'abarot*):

1. Urban: These were closer to cities, where most of the immigrants then worked.
2. Mixed: In these cases, people either worked in cities or in agriculture.
3. Agricultural: The immigrants worked mostly in farming.
4. Independent: These *ma'abarot* were intended from the start to develop into cities, such as Yeruham or Kiryat Shmona.

Mordechai Naor, *Sefer Haaliyot: Mea Shana ve Od shel Aliya ve klita* [The Book of Aliyot: One Hundred Years and More of Aliya and Absorption] (Tel Aviv: Ministry of Defense, 1991), 133–134.

28. Lissak, *Mass Immigration*, 28.

29. Moshe Lissak's breakdown of Israeli settlement policy for immigrants during the mass immigration is as follows:

1. May 1948–mid 1950: Immigrant camps
2. Mid 1950–mid 1952: *Maabarot* (transit camps)
3. Mid 1952–mid 1954: Plateau of Aliya—beginning of organized absorption
4. August 1954–mid 1956: "From the Boat to the Village"

Ibid., 24.

30. Ibid., 32.

31. Like in the case of Shaar Ha'aliya, there is—to date—no public, state remembrance of the transit camps (*maabarot*) although there has been, for a long time, some discussion of opening a ma'abara museum. The classic literary works that first captured the hardships of life in the transit camps are the works of Shimon Balas (*The Maabara*, 1964), Sami Michael (*Shavim ve Shavim Yoter*, 1974), and Eli Amir. Orit Bashkin's *Impossible Exodus* is a recent publication that—vividly and

in careful detail—portrays the extreme difficulty of life in the transit camps. See Bashkin, *Impossible Exodus*.

32. Zeev Tzahor, "Ben-Gurion's Attitude toward the *Gola* (Diaspora) and Aliyah," in *Kibbutz galuyot: Ha-aliyah le-Eretz Yisrael, mitos u-metzi'ut* [Ingathering of exiles: Aliyah to the Land of Israel, myth and reality], ed. Dvora Hacohen (Jerusalem: Zalman Shazar Center for Jewish History, 1998), 132.

33. George L. Mosse explains, "Nordau constantly used the phrase 'recapturing the dignity of the Jew' in his Zionist writings. This meant creating, as Nordau put it, deep-chested, powerfully built and keen-eyed men. A new type of Jew must be created who could end the threat of decadence among the Jews. The new Jew who would emerge from the wreckage of the diaspora symbolized the regeneration of the Jewish people" (George L. Mosse, "Max Nordau, Liberalism and the New Jew," *Journal of Contemporary History* 27, no. 4 [October 1992]: 567).

34. Shlomo Avineri, *The Making of Modern Zionism: The Intellectual Origins of the Jewish State* (New York: Basic Books, 1981), 154.

35. See "Muscle Jewry," in *Max Nordau to His People* [in Hebrew], ed. Benzion Netanyahu (Tel Aviv: Hotzaa Medinit, 1937); Mosse, "Max Nordau"; Anita Shapira, "Anti-Semitism and Zionism," *Modern Judaism* 15, no. 3 (October 1995): 215–232; Meira Weiss, *The Chosen Body* (Stanford: Stanford University Press, 2002). Tara Zahra discusses the Zionist hopes for transformation in *The Great Departure: Mass Migration from Eastern Europe and the Making of the Free World* (New York: Norton, 2016), 79.

36. Nadav Davidovitch and Rhona Seidelman, "Herzl's Altneuland: Zionist Utopia, Medical Science and Public Health," *Korot: The Israel Journal of the History of Medicine and Science* 17 (2003–2004): 1–21.

37. See Theodor Herzl, *Altneuland: Old-New Land*, trans. Paula Arnold (Haifa, Israel: Haifa, 1960); Davidovitch and Seidelman, "Herzl's Altneuland"; Weiss, *The Chosen Body*.

38. See Ari Barell, *Engineer King: David Ben-Gurion, Science and Nation Building* [in Hebrew] (Sde Boker, Israel: Sde Boker Research Institute for the Study of Israel and Zionism, 2014); Ari Barell, "Ha manheeg, ha madanim ve ha milchama: David Ben-Gurion ve hakamat heyil ha mada" [Leader, Scientists and War: David Ben-Gurion and the Establishment of the Science Corps], *Yisrael* 15 (2009): 67–92; Ari Barell, "Leviathan ve ha academia: haim haya nisayon lehaalim et ha universita ha ivrit beshnoteyha a rishonot shel midinat yisrael?," [Leviathan and Academia: Was There an Attempt to Nationalize the Hebrew University in the Early Years of the State of Israel?] *Tarbut Democratit* 13 (2011): 7–59; Shifra Shvarts, *The Workers' Health Fund in Eretz Israel: Kupat Holim, 1911–1937* (Rochester, N.Y.: University of Rochester Press, 2002).

39. European Christian Mission Hospitals first opened in 1838. These hospitals gave free treatment that still came at a cost to the Muslim and Jewish patients: while receiving treatment, they were forced to listen to teachings from the Christian gospel. And then—largely in response to, and out of fear from, the Christian medical proselytization—the local Jewish community finally accepted an offer from the philanthropist Moshe Montefiore to open a Jewish clinic with a Jewish doctor in 1854. Headed by Dr. Shimon Frankel, a German-Jewish doctor who was closely tied to ultra-Orthodox Haredi Jews, this was the first Jewish clinic that opened in Jerusalem, in 1854. Then from 1854 to 1902, five Jewish hospitals opened in Jerusalem, mostly as a result of conflicts in the different Jewish communities and the desire to have a hospital that better responded to the needs of the particular communities. These hospitals were Rothschild, Bikur Holim, Misgav Ledach, Shaarei Tzedek, and Ezrat Nashim. For the history of the first Jewish doctors and hospitals in Jerusalem, see Shifra Shvarts, "Hospital Wars" [in Hebrew], *Et Mol* 27, no. 2 (2001/2). On the history of Palestinian health care, see Nira Reiss, *The Health Care of the Arabs in Israel (Westview Special Studies on the Middle East)* (Boulder, Colo.: Westview, 1991); Sandra Sufian, "Arab Health Care during the British Mandate, 1920–1947," in *Separate and Cooperate, Cooperate and Separate: The Disengagement of the Palestine Health Care System from Israel and Its Emergence as an Independent System*, ed. Tamara Barnea and Rafiq Husseini (Westport, Conn.: Praeger, 2002), 9–31.

40. *Linat Tzedek* is a tradition of nighttime watch over the ill to ensure that they are not alone, while *bikur holim* is the charitable act of visiting the ill. To understand how these traditions were incorporated in Jewish health care in Palestine, see Shvarts, *The Workers' Health Fund*.

41. These physicians took the place previously held by traditional healers. Later, in what is known as the "fifth *Aliya*," numerous German physicians settled in the Jewish *Yishuv* in Palestine, thus significantly contributing to the persistence of European-trained health care workers. See Shvarts, "Hospital Wars."

42. The American approach gained a strong foothold primarily through the works of Hadassah, the philanthropical Women's Zionist Organization of America. Hadassah first began its work in medicine and public health in Palestine of the early twentieth century. For the history of Hadassah's involvement in Israeli health care, see Shifra Shvarts and Theodore M. Brown, "Kupat Holim, Dr. Isaac Max Rubinow and the American Zionist Medical Unit's Experiment to Establish Health Care Services in Palestine 1918–1923," *Bulletin of the History of Medicine* 72, no. 1 (1998): 28–46; Shifra Shvarts and Zipora Shehory-Rubin, *Hadassah for the Health of the People—the Health Education Mission of Hadassah: The American Zionist Women in the Holy Land* [in Hebrew] (Tel Aviv: Dekel Academic, 2012).

43. Sachlav Stoler-Liss, "'Mothers Birth the Nation': The Social Construction of Zionist Motherhood in Wartime in Israeli Parents' Manuals," *Nashim: A Journal of Jewish Women's Studies and Gender Issues* 6 (Fall 2003): 104–118.

44. Weiss, *The Chosen Body*.

45. On the immigration and absorption process of Holocaust survivors in Israel, see Hanna Yablonka, *Survivors of the Holocaust* (London: Macmillan, 1999).

46. Shaw and Capa, *Report on Israel*, 33.

47. On the concept of the "melting pot," see Lissak, *Mass Immigration*. For a more critical analysis, see Zvi Zameret, *Across a Narrow Bridge: Shaping the Education System During the Great Aliya* [in Hebrew] (Sde Boker, Israel: Ben-Gurion University of the Negev Press, 1997); Nadav Davidovitch and Shifra Shvarts, "Health and Hegemony: Preventive Medicine, Immigration and the Israeli Melting Pot," *Israel Studies* 9, no. 2 (2004): 150–179; Rakefet Zalashik, *History of Psychiatry in Palestine and Israel, 1882–1960* [in Hebrew] (Tel Aviv: Hakibbutz Hameuhad, 2008); Weiss, *The Chosen Body*.

48. Henrietta Dahan-Kalev, "You're So Pretty—You Don't Look Moroccan," *Israel Studies* 6, no. 1 (2001): 1–13. Aziza Khazoom refers to it as "Ashkenazification." She described this process as requiring "that Arabic Jews be marginalized within, but not excluded from, the economic and physical cores" (Aziza Khazzoom, "Did the Israeli State Engineer Segregation? On the Placement of Jewish Immigrants in Development Towns in the 1950s," *Social Forces* 84, no. 1 [September 2005]: 115–134).

49. CZA, AK 456/4, "Introduction" from Report on Shaar Ha'aliya, 10.8.52.

50. There was a section for the statistical department, Kupat Holim, and a general comments section for the use of the camp administration. CZA, AK 456/2, Administrative Report #7, 30.4.50.

51. CZA, AK 456/5.

52. CZA, AK 456/3, Administrative Report #19, 20.2.51; CZA, AK 456/3, Administrative Report #24, 30.4.51.

53. CZA, AK 456/8, Memories of Shaar Ha'aliya Written by Reznik, after March 1962; CZA, AK 456/3, Administrative Report #19, 20.2.51; CZA, AK 456/2, Exchange of Letters of Complaint and Weisberger's Response, 8.50.

54. CZA, AK 456/5, "Personal Equipment Card" and "Temporary Card."

55. Although the procedure was occasionally adjusted over the years, the main components of the processing system appear to have been constant: (1) reception and registration, (2) finding and settling into accommodations in the camp, (3) medical examinations, (4) customs declarations, (5) army arrangements, and (6) final housing assignments. These were the bureaucratic stages that had to be completed before the new immigrants were free to leave the camp for their permanent lodgings throughout the country (CZA, AK 456/5, "Tor Habikoret").

56. "Behitarvut hamishtara yatzu keh-2000 *olim* le ma'abarot" [2,000 *Olim* left for *ma'abarot* with police intervention], *Maariv*, August 8, 1951; "Bekoach mishtara maavirim *olim* meh *Shaar Ha'aliya* leh ma'abarot" [*Olim* are being transferred from *Shaar Ha'aliya* to *ma'abarot* through police force], *Al Hamishmar*, August 8, 1951.

57. Yehuda Weisberger, *Shaar Ha'aliya: The Diary of the Mass Aliya, 1947–1957* [in Hebrew] (Jerusalem: Bialik Institute, 1985), 64–65.

58. The person's cabin or tent number was recorded on their personal camp card, but there were still cases of people getting lost and of being unable to identify or find the tent or cabin they had been assigned. CZA, AK 456/8, Memories of Shaar Ha'aliya Written by Reznik, after March 1962.

59. "Ehad hamakeer shloshmeot ve hamishim elef" [One who knows 350,000], *Amar*, 1.4.56.

60. Rhona Seidelman, interview with D., 10.11.05. This interview was conducted as part of a research project directed by Prof. Shifra Shvarts, the Israel Science Foundation, 1217/04.

61. CZA, AK 456/8, Memories of Shaar Ha'aliya Written by Reznik, after March 1962.

62. Avraham Harman Institute of Contemporary Jewry, Oral History Division (hereafter OHD), (21), 38, 18; Hacohen, *Immigrants in Turmoil*, 289–291. Reuven Amoni, "Beshaari *Haaliya*" [At the gates of *Aliya*], *Davar*, September 18, 1950; Hacohen, *Immigrants in Turmoil*, 289–291; Weisberger, *Shaar H'aliya*, 75; CZA, AK 456/8, Memories of *Shaar Ha'aliya* Written by Reznik, after March 1962.

63. OHD, (210), 42.

64. CZA, AK 456/6, "Shaar Ha'aliya Facts and Figures," 1.4.55.

65. CZA, AK 456/1, "Movement of Immigrants through the Shaar Ha'aliya Processing Camp," 1.10.53–31.3.54.

66. The exact numbers are 77,245 from Iraq; 63,230 from Romania; 46,433 from Poland; 19,673 from Turkey; and 18,303 from Persia. The 69,743 North Africans included communities from Egypt, Libya, Tunisia, Algeria, and Morocco. Almost 40,000 families came through Shaar Ha'aliya. There were around 25,000 elderly people above the age of 60. Many others (close to 11,000) were what was listed as "family remnants, [. . .] the war's tragic yield" (CZA, AK 456/6, "Shaar Ha'aliya Facts and Figures," 1.4.55).

More than 300,000 immigrants to Israel from 1949 to 1954 did not go through Shaar Ha'aliya. This number includes approximately 100,000 people who came before Shaar Ha'aliya opened; 35,422 Yemenite immigrants who arrived in 1949 but did not go through Shaar Ha'aliya; and 22,000 to 42,000 people who went through Shaar Ha'aliya Bet. Of the remaining number, some may have gone to live with relatives, some may have been sick and immediately hospitalized, and others may have had their own financial resources and simply gone to live on their own accord. Moreover, there were certainly people who simply managed to avoid or flee Shaar Ha'aliya.

67. Theft: Amoni, *"Beshaarei Ha'aliya"*; CZA, AK 456/8, Memories of Shaar Ha'aliya Written by Reznik, after March 1962. Violence: "*Ehad hamakeer shloshmeot ve hamishim elef*"; Rhona Seidelman interview with C. C., 15.11.05. This interview was conducted as part of a research project directed by Prof. Shifra Shvarts, the Israel Science Foundation, 1217/04; Prostitution: Israel State Archives (hereafter ISA), 79/42 2295/1–ל, Police Report, 17.10.50.

68. CZA, AK 456/2, Administrative Report #7, 30.4.50.

69. CZA, AK 456/5, "Temporary Card"; Rhona Seidelman interview with E. S., 27.9.05; Rhona Seidelman interview with S. S., 27.9.05. These interviews were conducted as part of a research project directed by Prof. Shifra Shvarts, the Israel Science Foundation, 1217/04.

70. CZA, AK 456/3, Report on Employees' Meals, 5.6.49.

71. Boris Carmi, *Photographs from Israel*, ed. Alexandra Nocke (Munich: Prestel, 2004), 27; CZA, AK 456/2, "Camp Conditions" Letter to Editor, *Jerusalem Post* [in English], undated.

72. On food being unsuited to the various culinary traditions, see CZA, AK 456/1, Letter of Complaint, Dr. Berman, 2.2.51. Complaint about food at Shaar Ha'aliya: CZA, AK 456/1, Letter of Complaint, by J. O. [in English], 7.8.51. On wasted food: Weisberger, *Shaar Ha'aliya*, 75.

73. The most common explanation for why immigrants would not have left Shaar Ha'aliya was that they objected to the permanent residences they had been assigned by the Jewish Agency. The most common interpretation for why they had not left was that they preferred the sheltered existence in the camp (where they didn't have to work and were given free food) to subsisting independently outside Shaar Ha'aliya. These are explanations and interpretations given by camp administrators and not the immigrants themselves.

74. CZA, AK 456/2, Administrative Order #7, 30.4.50; CZA, AK 456/3, Administrative Order #44, 24.3.52.

75. Shaw and Capa, *Report on Israel*; CZA, AK 456/6, "*Shaar Le Aliya oh Mahaneh Hesger?*" (A gate for *Aliya* or a quarantine?), *Haolam Hazeh*, 31.03.51. On the line, see Rhona Seidelman, "Encounters in an Israeli Line: Shaar Ha'aliya, March 1950," *AJS Perspectives*, Fall 2014, http://perspectives.ajsnet.org/the-peoples-issue/encounters-in-an-israeli-line-shaar-ha-aliyah-march-1950/.

76. Amoni, *"Beshaarey Ha'aliya"*; CZA, AK 456/1, Letter to Editor by J. O., *Jerusalem Post*, July 1951; CZA, AK 456/1, Letter of Complaint, 8.50.

77. CZA, AK 456/3, Article on Shaar Ha'aliya in *Jewish Agency Digest*, March 1950. Many of the Shaar Ha'aliya staff members were themselves immigrants, although there are currently no numbers available for exactly how many were immigrants or what their countries of origin were.

78. CZA, AK 456/3, Administrative Report #39, 14.12.51.

79. Weisberger, *Shaar Ha'aliya*, 70.

80. Sick funds (*Kupot Holim*) are Israeli medical insurance organizations. The first sick fund began to operate in Palestine in 1913. It was established by Labor Zionists in response to the medical needs of their communities. By the time the state was established in 1948, there were four such funds in existence. For more on the history of Israel's sick funds, see Shvarts, *The Workers' Health Fund*.

81. CZA, AK 456/8, Report of "The Committee for the Study of New Immigrants and Their Absorption." April 1950; Interview with Dr. Hanna Szybuk, OHD, (210), 128, February 8, 1993; CZA, AK 456/3, Rundown of Illnesses at Shaar Ha'aliya, 1949–1954; CZA, AK 456/1, Report to Giora Josephtal on TB Treatment at Shaar Ha'aliya in 1949.

82. For a description of the minograph, see Clement F. Batelli, "Youth Interest High in War against Tuberculosis," *Health* 73, no. 6 (June 1946).

83. ISA, file 4251/23–57/3 ג, Report of Immigrant Health Services on Shaar Ha'aliya, 17.4.53.

84. Rhona Seidelman, S. Ilan Troen, and Shifra Shvarts, "'Healing' the Bodies and Souls of Immigrant Children: The Ringworm and Trachoma Institute, Shaar Ha'aliya, Israel 1952–1960," *Journal of Israeli History* 29, no. 2 (2010): 191–211.

85. CZA, AK 456/2, Report on Number of Immigrants Who Entered and Left Shaar Ha'aliya, 23.5.56. The attention given to the treatment of trachoma and ringworm, as well as improved hygiene and sanitation, had greatly diminished the incidence of these diseases in the prestate Jewish community in Palestine (*Yishuv*). Zipora Shehory-Rubin and Shifra Shvarts, "'*Hadassah' le-vri'ut ha-am: Pe'ilutah ha-bri'utit ha-hinukhit shel 'Hadassah' be-Eretz Yisrael bi-tkufat ha-mandat ha-briti*" ["Hadassah" for the health of the people: The health education work of "Hadassah" in Eretz Israel during the British Mandate] (Jerusalem: Ha-Sifriyah ha-Tziyonit, 2003), 90, 95.

With the mass immigration, the cases of these diseases once again grew in number. The decision to designate a separate area of Shaar Ha'aliya as a ringworm and trachoma institute touched upon some of the state's most fundamental concerns: immigration, health, and children. According to historian Avi Picard, "the heavy burden on health services, the deterioration of health conditions in Israel due to epidemics and infectious disease, and the dire economic straits led, beginning in 1952, to a policy of selective immigration" (Avi Picard, "Immigration, Health and

Social Control: Medical Aspects of the Policy Governing *Aliyah* from Morocco and Tunisia, 1951–54," *Journal of Israeli History* 22, no. 2 [Autumn 2003]: 33–34).

86. Kenneth F. Kiple, ed., *The Cambridge World History of Human Disease* (Cambridge: Cambridge University Press, 1993), 898; Thomas Lathrop Stedman, ed., *A Reference Handbook of the Medical Sciences* (New York: William Wood, 1917), 107.

87. Kiple, *The Cambridge World History*, 731; Baruch Modan et al., "Radiation-Induced Head and Neck Tumors," *Lancet* 303 (February 23, 1974): 277–279.

88. Stedman, *Reference Handbook of the Medical Sciences*, 203; Kiple, *Cambridge World History of Human Disease*, 735.

89. I discuss this more fully in Seidelman, Troen, and Shvarts, "'Healing' the Bodies and Souls."

90. Shannen K. Allen and Richard D. Semba, "The Trachoma 'Menace' in the United States, 1897–1960," *History of Ophthalmology* 47, no. 5 (September–October 2002): 501; Alan M. Kraut, *Silent Travellers: Germs, Genes and the Immigrant Menace* (Baltimore: Johns Hopkins University Press, 1994), 275–276.

91. "When the selective immigration policy and the plans to focus on *aliyah* from North African were approved, the Health Ministry and the Immigration Department reached a new agreement. In exchange for having its people put in charge of overseeing *aliyah* preparations in North Africa, the Ministry allowed a small number of ringworm patients (150 per month) to immigrate and be treated in Israel. A camp for ringworm and trachoma patients was set up at Sha'ar ha-Aliyah" (Seidelman, Troen, and Shvarts, "Healing the Bodies and Souls," 42).

92. CZA, AK 456/3, Report to Histadrut on Shaar Ha'aliya Activity, 18.2.55.

93. CZA, AK 456/3, Weisberger Report to Zionist Congress, 28.12.55.

94. CZA, AK 456/3, Letter from Dr. Chaim Sheba, 18.12.51.

95. Ibid.

96. CZA, AK 456/3, Report on Ringworm and Trachoma Institute, 8.7.52.

97. The precise number of people treated at the center is not clear. A 1956 document listed 5,487 cases treated for ringworm, as of 1952, and 2,715 for trachoma (CZA, AK 456/2, Report on Number of *Olim* Who Entered and Left Shaar Ha'aliya, 23.5.56). Modan and his coauthors put the number of immigrant children irradiated in Israel for ringworm in 1949–1960 at 17,000 (Modan et al., "Radiation-Induced Head and Neck Tumors," 277). However, Modan's figures also include the other smaller treatment centers in Tel Hashomer and Jerusalem while also taking into consideration the years before the Shaar Ha'aliya center opened. An article marking the closing of Shaar Ha'aliya in 1962 reported that 12,000 children had been treated at the ringworm and trachoma institute, but they do not specify how many had been treated for each disease (Rafael Bashan, "Kol Adam Hamishi Baaretz Yashav Kahn" [Every fifth person in the country sat here], *Ma'ariv*,

February 9, 1962). This figure is supported by the data in a table from the files of Yehuda Weisberger—director of Shaar Ha'aliya from 1949 to 1957—which tracks the number of children who went through the center from 1952 to 1955, listing approximately 8,000 children in these three years alone (CZA, AK 456/3, Handwritten Chart Titled "Ringworm").

98. CZA, AK 456/3, Report on Ringworm and Trachoma Institute, 8.7.52.

99. CZA, AK 456/2, WIZO Booklet [in English], August 1952.

100. CZA, AK 456/3, Report on Ringworm and Trachoma Institute, 8.7.52.

101. CZA, AK 456/3, Report to Histadrut on Shaar Ha'aliya Activity, 18.8.55; CZA, AK 456/6, Undated Report on Sha'ar ha-Aliyah activity, probably from 1954/55.

102. CZA, AK 456/1, Administrative Order #61, 16.8.53.

103. CZA, AK 456/1, Newspaper Article on Purim in the Ringworm and Trachoma Institute, undated.

104. "Cochin Newcomers Celebrate at Camp," *Jerusalem Post*, April 8, 1955.

105. CZA, AK 456/1, Report on Ringworm and Trachoma Institute, 8.7.52.

106. CZA, AK 456/3, Letter from Dr. Chaim Sheba, 18.12.51.

107. CZA, AK 456/2, "Shaar Ha'aliya Is Four," 26.3.53.

108. CZA, AK 456/6, Report in Weisberger File.

109. This link between health care, nation building, and socialization of children was a tradition that had already been rooted in the prestate *Yishuv*. See Dafna Hirsch, *"We Are Here to Bring the West": Hygiene Education and Culture Building in the Jewish Society of Palestine during the British Mandate Period* (Sde Boker, Israel: Ben-Gurion Research Institute for the Study of Israel and Zionism, 2014); Dafna Hirsch, "'Interpreters of the Occident to the Awakening Orient': The Jewish Public Health Nurse in Mandate Palestine," *Comparative Studies in Society and History* 50, no. 1 (2008): 227–255. To better understand the Zionist dedication to mother-infant health care with its roots in Ottoman Palestine, see Shifra Shvarts, "The Development of Mother and Infant Welfare Centers in Israel, 1854–1954," *Journal of the History of Medicine and Allied Sciences* 55, no. 4 (2000): 398–425.

110. CZA, AK 456/2, WIZO Booklet [in English], 8.52.

111. CZA, AK 456/3, Report on Ringworm and Trachoma Institute, 8.7.52.

112. "The hair was cut down to a level of 0.5 cm. and the scalp was divided into five fields, each being irradiated on one out of five consecutive days. The irradiation was done at three medical centres. . . . A temporary sterile cap was put on for eighteen to twenty-one days. Subsequently a cap of colophonium and wax was put on the head and taken off immediately after the wax had hardened, leading to a complete epilation of the hair. Some of the children were recalled for a second and even third course of treatment because of a relapse" (Modan et al., "Radiation-Induced Head and Neck Tumors," 277).

113. ISA, file 57/3 4251/23-ג, Letter in Response to a Complaint Made by Weisberger, 23.7.56.

114. This text is from the controversial documentary *Yaldei ha-gazezet* [*The Ringworm Children*] (see chapter 4). Here, there are in fact three testimonies that are interwoven to create one voice that expresses the similarity of the experience for different people. (English translation taken from movie subtitles.)

115. Sachlav Stoler-Liss, "Hadrakhah ve-kidum bri'ut be-hevrot rav tarbutiyot: Ha-mikreh shel ha-aliyah ha-gedolah le-Yisrael, 1949–1956" [Health promotion and health education in multicultural societies: The case of Israeli mass immigration, 1949–1956] (PhD diss., Ben-Gurion University of the Negev, 2006), 205.

116. Rhona Seidelman interview with D. N., October 9, 2005. This interview was conducted as part of a research project directed by Prof. Shifra Shvarts, the Israel Science Foundation, 1217/04.

117. Eli Amir, *Tarnegol kaparot* [*Scapegoat*] (Tel Aviv: Am Oved, 1990), 19.

118. David Belahsan and Asher Nehemias, *The Ringworm Children* (Israel: 2003).

119. This issue arose in the discussion that followed the screening of the movie *Yaldei ha-gazezet* [*The Ringworm Children*] at the Tel Aviv Cinematheque.

120. Kraut, *Silent Travellers*, 275–276.

121. Charles Rosenberg, "Disease in History: Frames and Framers," *Milbank Quarterly* 67, no. 1 (1989): 10.

122. The others included a Hadassah clinic in Jerusalem; the Tel Hashomer hospital; a Kupat Holim (Histadrut Sick Fund) clinic in Tel Aviv; a Hadassah clinic on Balfour Street in Tel Aviv; and a treatment center in Tiberias. Arab children were treated for ringworm at Rambam hospital in Haifa and, as of 1956, in Nazareth. Moreover, patients could also seek treatment from private physicians throughout Israel. See Seidelman, Shvarts, and Troen, "'Healing' the Bodies and Souls," 197.

123. CZA, AK 456/3, Report to Histadrut on Shaar Ha'aliya Activity, 18.2.55; CZA, AK 456/6, Undated Report on Shaar Ha'aliya Activity, probably from 1954/55. Although there is evidence to suggest that some Israeli-born children were sent to Shaar Ha'aliya for ringworm treatment (Shifra Shvarts interview with E. F., Israel Science Foundation, 1217/04), these would only have been cases where the parents had immigrated after 1948 and the child was born during the mass immigration. As a result, although the child would have in fact been Israeli-born, he or she would still have been strongly associated with the mass immigration. Children of "old-timers" who had ringworm tended to be treated in various local clinics run by their respective health care funds.

124. "Raeiti ve Shamati: Shaar Ha'aliya—machaneh ripui" [I saw and heard: "Shaar Ha'aliya"—healing camp], *Ha'aretz*, May 29, 1955.

125. On Shaar Ha'aliya Bet, see CZA, AK 456/3, Untitled Document Written after 1954; and CZA, AK 456/1, "Distribution of the Aliya from Ports of Arrival," 1.4.51–12.8.54. While one document suggests that twenty-two thousand people went through Shaar Ha'aliya Bet (CZA, AK 456/3, Untitled Document from Weisberger's Files, Written after 1954), another document claims that the figure was actually forty-two thousand (CZA, AK 456/1, "Distribution of the *Aliya* from Ports of Arrival," 1.4.51–12.8.54).

126. CZA, AK 456/3, List of Immigrants to Shaar Ha'aliya. See table 1.

127. CZA, AK 456/3, Letter from Mapai Cell in Shaar Ha'aliya to Mapai Office, Tel Aviv, 23.3.51; CZA, AK 456/6, Shaar Ha'aliya "Facts and Figures," 1.4.55.

128. CZA, AK 456/6, Report on Changes in Shaar Ha'aliya Administration, 18.2.55.

129. Rafael Bashan, "Kol Adam Hamishi Baaretz Yashav Kahn" [Every fifth person in the country sat here], *Ma'ariv*, February 9, 1962.

CHAPTER 2 — STRUCTURE

1. Sylvia Meltzer interview, Avraham Harman Institute of Contemporary Jewry, Oral History Division (hereafter OHD), (210), 141, 1993.

2. Leviticus 13:45.

3. Leviticus 14:19.

4. James A. Diamond explains that Maimonides considered leprosy to be a "sign and wonder," brought on by wicked speech. The leprosy, a warning for the slanderer to change, "began on walls, spread to furniture, then to clothing, and finally to the physical person." If the person failed to repent as the stages of leprosy escalated, he would finally be forced to dwell apart. This seclusion would force the person to forsake evil speech; by having no one to converse with, the person would be compelled to silence. James A. Diamond, "Maimonides on Leprosy: Illness as Contemplative Metaphor," *Jewish Quarterly Review* 96, no. 1 (Winter 2006): 95–122.

However, in his discussion on how Jewish ethics would approach the involuntary confinement of noncompliant patients with active tuberculosis, Fred Rosner has convincingly used the biblical passages on leprosy to illustrate a scenario in which it is permissible to set aside individual rights "to protect the health and welfare of society." Rosner has refocused the biblical passage onto the benefits to the community, rather than solely the curative and punitive experience for the individual. Rosner suggests that the forced separation of the leper safeguarded the public's health. Moreover, his article sheds light on the central conflict inherent to the concept of quarantine: the rights of the group versus the rights of the individual. Fred Rosner, "Involuntary Confinement for Tuberculosis Control: The Jewish View," *Mount Sinai Journal of Medicine* 63, no. 1 (January 1996): 44–48.

5. George Rosen, *A History of Public Health* (New York: MD, 1958), 64–65.

6. Ibid., 67. For a classic literary work on the Black Plague, see Giovanni Boccaccio, *The Decameron* (New York: Dell, 1976). For a later account, see the depiction of the last great plague of London in 1772 in Daniel Defoe, *A Journal of the Plague Year* (London: Penguin Books, 2003).

7. Rosen, *History of Public Health*, 69.

8. Paul Kelton, "Avoiding the Smallpox Spirits: Colonial Epidemics and Southeastern Indian Survival," *Ethnohistory* 51, no. 1 (Winter 2004): 58.

9. Ibid., 59.

10. Ibid., 61.

11. In exploring how the contact with Europeans resulted in devastating illness and death among Native Americans, Alan M. Kraut explains that Europeans were not quarantined by the Native Americans because "use of such a preventive presupposes awareness of risk." Although isolation and quarantine traditions did exist in Native American culture, there were cases in which Native American tradition called for close contact with their sick and quarantine would have been seen as a cruel and "undeserved ostracism" (Alan M. Kraut, *Silent Travellers: Germs, Genes and the Immigrant Menace* [Baltimore: Johns Hopkins University Press, 1994], 12, 15).

12. Michael W. Dols, "The Leper in Islamic Society," *Speculum* 58, no. 4 (1983): 907–908.

13. Ibid., 910.

14. Ibid., 911.

15. *Encyclopedia of the Black Death*, s.vv. "The Prophet Muhammed," "Justinian, Plague of (First Plague Pandemic)," accessed January 5, 2018, https://ou-primo.hosted.exlibrisgroup.com; Lester Little, *Plague and the End of Antiquity: The Pandemic of 541–750* (Cambridge: Cambridge University Press, 2008); Kyle Harper, *The Fate of Rome: Climate, Disease, and the End of an Empire* (Princeton: Princeton University Press, 2017).

16. *Encyclopedia of the Black Death*, s.v. "Islamic Civil Response to the Black Death."

17. In the preliminary remarks of Birsen Bilmus's book *Plague, Quarantine and Geopolitics in the Ottoman Empire* (Edinburgh: Edinburgh University Press, 2011), she presents an important discussion of this issue among scholars.

18. *Encyclopedia of the Black Death*, s.v. "Islamic Civil Response to the Black Death."

19. Ibid.

20. Dorothy Porter, *Health, Civilization and the State: A History of Public Health from Ancient to Modern Times* (London: Routledge, 1999), 140. Alan M. Kraut's

work also supports this claim. He shows the prevalence of the idea in nineteenth century America that disease was the fault of the people who were sick: "This melding of the miasmatic theory with a growing fear of contagia served to bind the cause of disease directly to the sufferer" (Kraut, *Silent Travellers*, 23).

21. David F. Musto, "Quarantine and the Problem of AIDS," *Milbank Quarterly* 64, supp. 1 (1986): 102.

22. Eugenia Tognotti, "Lessons from the History of Quarantine, from Plague to Influenza A," *Emerging Infectious Diseases* 19, no. 2 (February 2013): 256. For a discussion on both the policy and experience of Britain's nineteenth-century quarantine system, see Krista Maglen, "'The First Line of Defence': British Quarantine and the Port Sanitary Authorities in the Nineteenth Century," *Social History of Medicine* 15, no. 3 (2002): 414–428; Krista Maglen, "Quarantined: Exploring Personal Accounts of Incarceration in Australian and Pacific Quarantine Stations in the Nineteenth Century," *Journal of the Royal Australian Historical Society* 91, no. 1 (2005): 1–12.

23. Roy Porter, *The Greatest Benefit to Mankind: A Medical History of Humanity* (New York: W. W. Norton, 1997).

24. Nancy Tomes, *The Gospel of Germs: Men, Women and the Microbe in American Life* (Cambridge, Mass.: Harvard University Press, 1999), 254. This sense of confidence of physicians and scientists that infectious disease could become a concern of the past is evident with some of the earliest proponents of germ theory. Charles Rosenberg explains that once germ theory was proven, there was a sense that it would only be a matter of time before physicians understood all microorganisms. Charles Rosenberg, "Disease in History: Frames and Framers," *Milbank Quarterly* 67, no. 1 (1989): 8.

25. Two notable examples of the successful use of quarantine in late twentieth and early twenty-first centuries are the 2003 SARS epidemic and the 2014 outbreak of the Ebola virus. Severe quarantine measures were taken in order to end the spread of both of these diseases. In this way, they serve as examples of the successes of quarantine—it can still be both necessary and effective to stop the spread of disease. But as is often the case in the history of quarantine and the panic that can accompany epidemics, we can also find in these stories instances of forcible quarantine that were unnecessary, sometimes racist as well as violating. One of the most famous cases of panicked and unnecessary forcible quarantine in the United States during the 2014 Ebola pandemic was that of Kaci Hickox, a nurse from Texas who had traveled to Sierra Leone to work with Doctors without Borders during the Ebola outbreak. When she returned to the United States, Hickox was quarantined in the airport in New Jersey, though she had no signs that she had the virus. For more on Hickox's quarantine experience, see Kaci Hickox, "Her Story: UTA

Grad Isolated at New Jersey Hospital in Ebola Quarantine," *Dallas Morning News*, October 25, 2014.

26. CDC, "Quarantine and Isolation," accessed July 19, 2019, https://www.cdc.gov/quarantine/index.html.

27. Moshe Lissak refers to the camp as St. Lucas (Moshe Lissak, *The Mass Immigration in the Fifties: The Failure of the Melting Pot Policy* [in Hebrew] [Jerusalem: Bialik Institute, 1999], 25). In the article "Israel's First Year," *Illustrated*, August 27, 1949, Robert Capa refers to it as St. Luke. "Lucas" may have resulted from mishearing "Luke" in Hebrew and then misspelling it.

28. There were 122 preexisting buildings, and 134 new ones were added. Central Zionist Archive (hereafter CZA), AK 456/4, Report on Shaar Ha'aliya, 6.52.

29. CZA, AK 456/4, "Boundaries" in Report on Shaar Ha'aliya, 6.52. The one exception in which the internal barbed wire fence was retained was the boundary between the main camp and the smaller southern area that, in 1952, was turned into the Institute for the Treatment of Ringworm and Trachoma.

30. Ibid.

31. For a few examples, see Orit Rozin, *The Rise of the Individual in 1950s Israel: A Challenge to Collectivism* (Waltham, Mass.: Brandeis University Press, 2011); Dvora Hacohen, *Immigrants in Turmoil: The Great Wave of Immigration to Israel and Its Absorption, 1948–1953* [in Hebrew] (Jerusalem: Yad Yitzhak Ben Tzvi, 1994); Shifra Shvarts, *Health and Zionism: The Israeli Health Care System, 1948–1960* (Rochester, N.Y.: University of Rochester Press, 2008)

32. Hacohen, *Immigrants in Turmoil*, 187.

33. Shvarts, *Health and Zionism*, 158.

34. Rozin, *The Rise of the Individual*, cited in Orit Bashkin, *Impossible Exodus: Iraqi Jews in Israel* (Stanford: Stanford University Press, 2017), 68, 252.

35. Avi Picard, "Immigration, Health and Social Control: Medical Aspects of the Policy Governing *Aliyah* from Morocco and Tunisia, 1951–54," *Journal of Israeli History* 22, no. 2 (2003): 52.

36. Hanna Yablonka, *Survivors of the Holocaust* (London: Macmillan, 1999), 9.

37. Rozin, *Rise of the Individual in 1950s Israel*, 151; Michael A. Davies, "Health and Disease in Israel, 1948–1994," in *Health and Disease in the Holy Land: Studies in the History and Sociology of Medicine from Ancient Times to the Present*, ed. Manfred Waserman and Samuel S. Kottek (Lewiston, N.Y.: Edwin Mellen, 1996). As expressed by Dr. Avraham Sternberg, head of the Immigrant Health Services during the mass immigration, "The remnants of European Jewry comprised a complicated health problem because of the physical and mental suffering that they had experienced" (Avraham Sternberg, *A People Is Absorbed* [Tel Aviv: Hakibbutz Hameuhad, 1973], 21).

38. Picard, "Immigration, Health and Social Control," 34.

39. Theodor Grushka, *Health Services in Israel* (Jerusalem: Ministry of Health, 1968), 35.

40. Shifra Shvarts, Nadav Davidovitch, Rhona Seidelman, and Avishay Goldberg, "Medical Selection and the Debate over Mass Immigration in the New State of Israel (1948–1951)," *Canadian Bulletin for the History of Medicine* 22, no. 1 (2005): 12.

41. Picard, "Immigration, Health and Social Control," 34.

42. Sachlav Stoler-Liss, "Hadrakhah ve-kidum bri'ut be-hevrot rav tarbutiyot: Ha-mikreh shel ha-aliyah ha-gedolah le-Yisrael, 1949–1956" [Health promotion and health education in multicultural societies: The case of Israeli mass immigration, 1949–1956] (PhD diss., Ben-Gurion University of the Negev, 2006), 51.

43. Ibid., 54–70.

44. CZA, AK 456/3, "Classification of Diseases, 1949–1954." The low rate of polio was explained by Ireka Einav, who worked as a pediatric nurse in Shaar Ha'aliya: "We did not have many cases [of polio]. The cases that we had were diagnosed very early" (Ireka Einav, interviewed by Hava Ulman, OHD, [210], 135, March 1, 1993).

45. Stoler-Liss, "Hadrakhah ve-kidum bri'ut be-hevrot rav tarbutiyot" [Health promotion and health education in multicultural societies], 70.

46. Ibid. We know from Michael Davies that there were three epidemics in Israel during the mass immigration: malaria, tuberculosis, and polio (Davies, "Health and Disease," 448).

47. New immigrants received three months of free health insurance through the Labor-Zionist-affiliated General Sick Fund (Kupat Holim Clalit). At the end of the three months, they would then have to pay a small monthly fee, and they could choose to have their coverage through any one of the four existing (and competing) sick funds. Shvarts, *Health and Zionism*, 187.

48. According to Shvarts, the breakdown of hospitals was as follows: three public hospitals in Jerusalem (Misgav Ladah, Shaarei Zedek, and Bikur Holim) and one public psychiatric hospital (Ezrat Nahim), three hospitals run by the sick fund Kupat Holim Clalit (Belinson, Haemek, and the psychiatric hospital Geha), four Hadassah hospitals (Jerusalem, Tel Aviv, Haifa, and Tzfat), two birthing centers (Kupat Holim Clalit's center in Kfar Saba and Tel Aviv's municipal center at the Kiriya). There were also thirty-one private hospitals or nonprofit health organizations, small institutions that provided public services including care for mental health patients and people with disabilities. In these numbers, Shvarts has not included the hospitals that were in transition, such as British governmental or military hospitals that were run for a while after the establishment of the state but not specifically in May 1948. Shifra Shvarts, "The Birth of Israel Health Care

System—an American Mother and a Russian Father" (lecture, University of North Carolina, Chapel Hill, September 2000).

49. Shifra Shvarts, "International Health and Welfare Organizations in Israel: The Early Years," in *Katyn and Switzerland: Forensic Investigators and Investigations in Humanitarian Crises, 1920–2007* [in French and English], ed. Delphine Debons, Antoine Fleury, and Jean-François Pitteloud (Geneva: Georg, 2009), 325–334.

50. Ibid., 325.

51. Sternberg, *A People Is Absorbed*, 17.

52. Ibid., 20, 22, 38.

53. Ibid., 128.

54. The diseases listed as "quarantinable" in Israel at this time were smallpox and louse-borne typhus. Grushka writes, "During the period under review [1948–1965] no cases of quarantinable diseases were reported in the country nor were any registered in Israeli vessels" (*Health Services in Israel*, 109). See also Nissim Levy's discussion of quarantine in Israel at this time.

55. Thomas Lathrop Stedman, ed., *A Reference Handbook of the Medical Sciences* (New York: William Wood, 1917), 107.

56. CZA, AK 456/6, Letter from Weisberger to Kalman Levin, 9.11.50.

57. CZA, AK 456/3, Letter from Weisberger to PR Office, 28.2.51.

58. CZA, AK 456/8, Memories of Shaar Ha'aliya Written by Reznik, after March 1962.

59. It is not clear whether he had intended to push the boundaries in an attempt to test the guards and the Shaar Ha'aliya administration, but a complaint was filed and the guards were accused of beating the reporter. The police file denies that he was beaten, and Weisberger appears to have stood by the police report, submitting it as the official reply to *Davar*. CZA, AK 456/2, Police Report on *Davar* Reporter's Complaint, 3.12.50.

60. CZA, AK 456/8, "Absorption Pangs": Report of Committee for the Study of *Olim* and Their Absorption, 4.50.

61. Rafael Bashan, "Kol Adam Hamishi Baaretz Yashav Kahn" [Every fifth person in the country sat here], *Ma'ariv*, February 9, 1962.

62. This encounter is documented in Refael Sela, "Shaar Le Aliyah oh Mahaneh Hesger?" [A gate for *Aliya* or a quarantine?], *Haolam Hazeh*, May 31, 1951.

63. ISA, file 79/5 2177/38ל–, Report of General Investigation Department, Haifa Police, 26.11.50.

64. Bryan K. Roby, *The Mizrahi Era of Rebellion: Israel's Forgotten Civil Rights Struggle, 1948–1966* (Syracuse, N.Y.: Syracuse University Press, 2015); Orit Rozin, *A Home for All Jews: Citizenship, Rights, and National Identity in the New Israeli State* (Waltham, Mass.: Brandeis University Press, 2016); Bashkin, *Impossible Exodus*.

65. ISA, file 79/5 2177/38ל-, Report of General Investigation Department, Haifa Police. 26.11.50.

66. The camp administration tried different approaches to get people to leave. One was to deny subsidized food to people who stayed longer than the administration wanted them to (CZA, AK 456/2, Letter of Complaint to *Jerusalem Post*, by Y. L. M., 11.53). But the immigrants also fought this policy: In several cases, camp residents joined together to give portions of their own food to those who did not have any. This allowed people to stay on in the camp even as the administration tried to force them out. The other approach taken by the camp administration was forced evacuation: "Bekoach mishtara maavirim *olim* meh *Shaar Ha'aliya* leh ma'abarot" [*Olim* are being transferred from *Shaar Ha'aliya* to *ma'abarot* through police force], *Al Hamishmar*, August 8, 1951; "Behitarvut hamishtara yatzu keh-2000 *olim* le ma'abarot" [2,000 *Olim* left for *Ma'abarot* with police intervention], *Maariv*, August 9, 1951.

67. CZA, AK 456/2, A series of letters from 1953, including complaints about Shaar Ha'aliya that were sent to the newspaper the *Jerusalem Post*, notes from the Jewish Agency to Weisberger asking him to respond to the complaints and Weisberger's response; CZA, AK 456/3, Report on State of Shaar Ha'aliya from Mapai Representatives Working There, to Their Main Center in Tel Aviv, 23.5.51; ISA, 2177/38-ל, Shaar Ha'aliya Police File, 50–53.

68. CZA, AK 456/2, Letter of Complaint to *Jerusalem Post*, by Y. L. M. [in English], 11.53.

69. CZA, AK 456/2, Letter of Complaint from Immigrant, 18.9.1950.

70. CZA, AK 456/1, Letter from August 1951, Series of Documents between the Jewish Agency and Weisberger Regarding a Letter of Complaint about Shaar Ha'aliya from an Immigrant, Including a Copy of the Letter from the Immigrant.

71. CZA, AK 456/4, Survey of Shaar Ha'aliya Buildings and Property, 52. In his description of the hunger strike, Yehuda Weisberger wrote that there were three huts for TB patients. Yehuda Weisberger, *Shaar Ha'aliya: The Diary of the Mass Aliya, 1947–1957* [in Hebrew] (Jerusalem: Bialik Institute, 1985), 126.

72. Sternberg, *A People Is Absorbed*, 128.

73. Davies, "Health and Disease," 448.

74. Sternberg, *A People Is Absorbed*, 129.

75. Rhona Seidelman interview with S. H., October 23, 2005. This interview was conducted as part of a research project directed by Prof. Shifra Shvarts, the Israel Science Foundation, 1217/04.

76. This is an excellent example of how different the experience at Shaar Ha'aliya could have been for a person based on familiarity with languages and proximity

to the Ashkenazi elite. As we see here, having access to the languages of the people in positions of authority—in this case, the (presumably) Ashkenazi doctor—was critical. For this woman, language made the most important difference a mother could possibly imagine: having her child taken away from her or not.

77. CZA, AK 456/8, Booklet from Jewish Agency Public Relations Division, 1.50.

78. See, for example, Ella Shohat, "Sephardim in Israel: Zionism from the Standpoint of Its Jewish Victims," *Social Text*, no. 19/20 (Autumn 1988): 1–35; Yehuda Shenhav, *The Arab Jews: A Postcolonial Reading of Nationalism, Religion, and Ethnicity* (Stanford: Stanford University Press, 2006).

79. This situation firmly aligns with Orit Bashkin's conceptualization of resistance and her insistence that in this period so many acts—both big and small—were all part of "the victories in the daily and public battles to maintain public dignity" (Bashkin, *Impossible Exodus*).

80. Here, again, I turn to Bashkin's conceptualization of resistance to help underscore the significance of what was happening at Shaar Ha'aliya. She writes that resistance "came in many manners and forms. In my opinion, Iraqi mothers in transit camps who managed to get their children out of the cycle of poverty by working several jobs; teachers who organized classes and schools, without state permission; and Iraqi children who critiqued the lifestyle of the kibbutzim that hosted them, were no less heroic than those of the more organized groups of the Israeli Black Panthers in the 1970's. Perhaps they were even more so" (ibid., 11).

81. ISA, 79/42 2295/1–ל, Letter from Y. Sheffi to Absorption Department, 10.8.50.

82. ISA, file 79/5 2145/21–ל, Report on the Introduction of a Police Presence in *Shaar Ha'aliya*, 19.7.49; CZA, AK 456/1, Letter from Giora Josephtal, 4.7.49.

83. ISA, file 79/42 2295/1, Report on Shaar Ha'aliya Guards, 13.4.51.

84. In December 1949, after he had helped them arrange a Hanukah party for their unit, the police sent Yehuda Weisberger an effusive letter of thanks expressing their wish for the continuation of a positive relationship. However, these hopes appear to have been seriously disappointed.

85. ISA, file 79/42 2295/1–ל, Weisberger Report on Shaar Ha'aliya Police, 28.1.51.

86. ISA, file 79/42 2295/1–ל, Report from Shefi on Situation for Police at Shaar Ha'aliya, 28.2.51.

87. Ibid.

88. The problems encountered in the police force were not unlike those of many government bodies in the early years of the state, which were all very new and functioning quite tenuously. On the transition into statehood and the crystallization of these institutions, see Zvi Zameret and Hana Yablonka, eds., *The First Decade* [in Hebrew] (Jerusalem: Yad Yitzhak Ben-Tzvi, 1997); Ruth Kark, "Planning, Housing,

and Land Policy 1948–1952: The Formation of Concepts of Governmental Frameworks," in *Israel: The First Decade of Independence*, ed. S. Ilan Troen and Noah Lucas (Albany: State University of New York Press, 1995), 461–495.

89. ISA, file 79/42 2295/1–ל, Shefi Report on Situation for Police at Shaar Ha'aliya, 8.50.

90. Ibid.

91. CZA, AK 456/3, Report from Kalman Levin to Giora Josephtal, 24.8.50.

92. ISA, 79/42 2295/1–ל, Letter from Giora Josephtal to Y. Shefi, 1.9.50.

93. ISA, file 79/42 2295/1–ל, Nehmias Letter, 6.3.51.

94. ISA, file 79/42 2295/1–ל, Report on Situation for Guards at Shaar Ha'aliya, 13.4.51.

95. CZA, AK 456/4, "Boundaries" in Report on Shaar Ha'aliya, 6.52.

CHAPTER 3 — MEANING

1. K. Shabtai, "Shaar Ha'aliya Mishavea Letukinim" [Shaar Ha'aliya desperately needs repair], *HaDor*, April 8, 1951.

2. See Israel State Archives (hereafter ISA), file 79/42 2295/1–ל, Police Report on Shaar Ha'aliya Labeled Secret and Personal, 28.2.51; ISA, file 79/42 2295/1–ל, Report on Situation for Guards at Shaar Ha'aliya, 13.4.51.

3. The one important perspective that is not included in this chapter is that of the immigrants themselves, which is discussed instead in chapter 4. There are rich sources available that document the immigrants' reactions to Shaar Ha'aliya's fence, but they are almost all retrospectives. For that reason, I chose to include them as part of the discussion on historical remembrances.

4. *Encyclopedia Judaica*, 2nd ed., s.v. "Ruth Gruber"; "In Memoriam: Ruth Gruber," *Holocaust and Genocide Studies* 31, no. 1 (Spring 2017): 185; Ruth Gruber, *Ahead of Time: My Early Years as a Foreign Correspondent* (New York: Carroll & Graf, 2001); Ruth Gruber, *Inside of Time: My Journey from Alaska to Israel* (New York: Carroll & Graf, 2003).

5. The articles' full titles are as follows:

> "Sailing for the Promised Land (The Story of a Refugee Ship And the Last Lap to Israel)";
>
> "Refugees, on Voyage to Israel, Realize They Will Be Pioneers (Immigrants on the Atzmaut Are Prepared to Face Austerity and Hardships for Life of Hope)";
>
> "Aboard Refugee Ship for Israel No Comfort, But Spirits Are High";

"Aboard Refugee Ship for Israel A Wedding Adds Gayety to Trip (Couple Who Fled Hungary Are Married by Captain And Again by Rabbi in Ancient Rite)";

"Refugees' Landing in Israel: 'It's Our Land, It Belongs to Us' (Atzmaut's 1,700 Passengers Sing 'Hatikvah' As Ship Docks at Haifa, and They Disperse to Camps)"; and

Ruth Gruber, *The New York Herald Tribune*, August 7–11, 1949.

6. Raymond Cartier, "Israël: Étendue: Trois départements Mission: Résoudre dans le monde le problème juif," *Paris-Match*, August 13, 1949, 24–34. A translated summary of this article also appears in Weisberger's files. CZA, AK 456/1.

7. On Raymond Cartier and Cartierism, see Todd Shepherd, *The Invention of Decolonization: The Algerian War and the Remaking of France* (Ithaca, N.Y.: Cornell University Press, 2006). Shepherd writes of Cartier that he was a "well-known columnist for the incredibly popular photo-weekly *Paris-Match*, both (the man and the magazine) purveyors of blandly mainstream right-wing populism" (96).

8. Headlines declaring Capa to be one of the world's best photographers started appearing in the late 1930s. Richard Whelan, *Robert Capa: A Biography* (New York: Alfred A. Knopf, 1985), 151–157.

9. According to Richard Whelan, Capa is said to have left in in the midst of the 1948 war, after a dangerous encounter left him shaken: While taking photographs of the clash between the different Jewish fighting units at the *Altalena*, he was grazed by a bullet but—by chance—not injured. He packed his bags and booked a seat on the next flight from Tel Aviv to Paris. Ibid., 265.

10. Irwin Shaw and Robert Capa, *Report on Israel* (New York: Simon & Schuster, 1950).

11. Whelan, *Robert Capa*, 267–268; Alex Kershaw, *Blood and Champagne: The Life and Times of Robert Capa* (London: Macmillan, 2002), 213.

12. Whelan, *Robert Capa*, 267. Whelan recounts that Capa even considered settling down in Tel Aviv and encouraged his mother to think about moving there (269).

13. One quote that reinforces this idea is as follows: "Capa was always—throughout his entire career—primarily a photographer of *people*, and many of his pictures of war (even those taken in the midst of battle) are not so much chronicles of events as extraordinarily sympathetic and compassionate studies of people under extreme stress" (ibid., 105).

14. Kershaw, *Blood and Champagne*, 213.

15. Robert Capa, "Israel's First Year," *Illustrated*, August 27, 1949.

16. Whelan, *Robert Capa*, 267.

17. Ibid.

18. Ibid., 268.

19. Capa, "Israel's First Year," quoted in Whelan, *Robert Capa*, 267.

20. Shaw and Capa, *Report on Israel*.

21. I am intrigued by the idea that Gruber, Cartier, and Capa may all have encountered one another while they were at Shaar Ha'aliya, since their articles were all published in the same month.

22. Perhaps, as Jews, Gruber and Capa both had some degree of connection to the place. But of course, neither of them were Israeli, and neither of them chose to stay in Israel.

23. Yehuda Weisberger, *Shaar Ha'aliya: The Diary of the Mass Aliya, 1947–1957* [in Hebrew] (Jerusalem: Bialik Institute, 1985), 115.

24. Ibid., 71.

25. Ibid.

26. Central Zionist Archive (hereafter CZA), AK 456/1, Letter from Kalman Levin to Dr. Berman, 14.3.51.

27. Ibid.

28. CZA, AK 456/4, "Introduction" from Report on Shaar Ha'aliya, 10.8.52. An earlier report, from June 1952, conveyed the camp's purpose similarly: "The idea for a processing camp came in answer to two problems that the Absorption Department was considering in those days: how to turn the new immigrant into a citizen of Israel in only a few days, and how to protect the Yishuv from diseases that were likely to befall it as a result of this immigration" (CZA, AK 456/4, "Boundaries" in Report on Shaar Ha'aliya, 6.52).

29. A copy of this article can be found in Weisberger's archives. CZA, AK 456/2.

30. This is how Weisberger ended his letter: "Allow me to add that around two months ago there was a man from South America from among the immigrants who presented himself as a journalist and submitted a complaint to the administration that was comprised of almost all the aforementioned points, with the addition of a complaint of beatings the immigrants received from the clerks . . . Following an appropriate investigation a directive came from the Prime Minister's office to promptly transfer the complainant to an institute for the mentally ill" (CZA, AK 456/2, Letter from Weisberger to PR division, Absorption Department, Tel Aviv, 4.9.50).

31. Weisberger's position here is one that he took on other occasions. In a letter from Weisberger to the Absorption Department in Tel Aviv, September 4, 1950 (CZA, AK 456/2), he wrote that the quarantine was necessary "to protect the health of the Yishuv from contagious diseases from abroad." In a letter to Kalman Levin,

November 9, 1950, he wrote that "there was '[a] need to protect the country's residents from the danger of the diseases'" (CZA, AK 456/6). There was also the April 1950 report of the "Committee for the Study of Immigrants and their Absorption," of which Weisberger was a member, that similarly states that the medical examinations at Shaar Ha'aliya "reveal a large degree of sick people who are dangerous to the surroundings" (CZA, AK 456/8, "Absorption Pangs," Report of Committee for the Study of Immigrants and Their Absorption).

32. ISA, 79/42 2295/1–ל, Letter from Y. Sheffi to Absorption Department, 10.8.50.

33. Mary Douglas, *Purity and Danger: An Analysis of Pollution and Taboo* (London: Penguin Books, 1970), 125.

34. As articulated by Kraut, "knowing that the stigmatized victim is from another place brings with it the reassurance that one's own body and surroundings are inherently healthy and would remain so were it not for the presence of the stranger" (Alan M. Kraut. *Silent Travellers: Germs, Genes and the Immigrant Menace* [Baltimore: Johns Hopkins University Press, 1994], 26).

35. David F. Musto, "Quarantine and the Problem of AIDS," *Milbank Quarterly* 64, supp. 1 (1986): 98, 108.

36. Ben-Gurion Archives, Meetings File, 27.3.49, quoted in Zvi Zameret, "Ben-Gurion and Lavon: Two Standpoints on Absorption during the Great Wave of Immigration," in *Israel in the Great Wave of Immigration* [in Hebrew], ed. Dalia Ofer (Jerusalem: Yad Yitzhak Ben Tzvi, 1996), 77.

37. Shaw and Capa, *Report on Israel*, 33.

38. Ibid., 37.

39. Moshe Lissak, "Images of Immigrants: Stereotypes and Stigmatization in the Period of Mass Immigration to Israel in the 1950s" [in Hebrew] *Cathedra*, 43 (1987): 125.

40. Ibid., 127.

41. *Vatik*, while difficult to translate, can be understood as a resident who was no longer considered a new immigrant.

42. Meir Shalev, *The Blue Mountain* (New York: Harper Perennial, 1991), 22.

43. Avner Holtzman, "The Encounter between Newcomers and 'Oldtimers' as Reflected in Hebrew Fiction" [in Hebrew], in Ofer, *Israel in the Great Wave of Immigration*, xi.

44. Dan Horowitz and Moshe Lissak, *Trouble in Utopia: The Overburdened Polity of Israel* (Albany: State University of New York Press, 1989), 13.

45. "In contrast to the founding fathers, who turned their backs on the Jewish village of Eastern Europe, because of the degeneration they associated with it, the immigrants from Asia and Africa were at peace with their worlds as they had crystallized in the Diaspora [. . .] The identity of the immigrants from the Eastern

countries, which was strong and rooted, posed a threat to the Zionist ethos as a defining power" (Henriette Dahan-Kalev, "Israeli Identity—between New Immigrants and 'Oldtimers,'" in Ofer, *Israel in the Great Wave of Immigration*, 181).

See also the infamous series "I Was a New Immigrant for One Month" written by journalist Aryeh Gelblum in 1949. In these articles, Gelblum brought to the Israeli public a detailed account of the terrible conditions for people in Israel's immigrant camps while also displaying a deep prejudice, as evident in his disparaging depiction of immigrants from "North African and Arab" countries. These articles are a discussion of life in several different immigrant camps. They came out a few weeks after Shaar Ha'aliya opened. "Hodesh Yamim Hayiti Oleh Hadash" in Shimon Rubinstein, *The Full Collection of Articles Published by Aryeh Gelblum in "Haaretz" (13.4–6.5 1949) and the Responses to Aliya* [in Hebrew], illus. by Gerti Rubinstein (Jerusalem, 2001).

46. Moshe Lissak, *The Mass Immigration in the Fifties: The Failure of the Melting Pot Policy* [in Hebrew] (Jerusalem: Bialik Institute, 1999), 62.

47. Orit Rozin, "'Terms of Disgust': Hygiene and Parenthood of Immigrants from Moslem Countries as Viewed by Veteran Israelis in the 1950s" [in Hebrew], *Iyunim Bitkumat Israel* 12 (2002): 204, 218, 219, 237.

48. Haim Malka, *The Selection: Selection and Discrimination in the Aliya and Absorption of Moroccan and North African Jewry 1948–1956* [in Hebrew] (Tel Aviv: Tal, 1998)

49. Hanna Yablonka, *Survivors of the Holocaust* (London: Macmillan, 1999), 63–72.

50. Her book mentions numerous walls but Brown explains her decision to focus her analysis on United States / Mexico and Israel/Palestine because they are "the two largest, most expensive, and most notorious of the new walls" (Wendy Brown, *Walled States, Waning Sovereignty* [New York: Zone Books, 2010], 28).

51. Ibid., 27. Shaar Ha'aliya's smaller fence also has a place within Brown's analysis as part of the broader idea of a physical barrier.

52. "Political walls have always spectacularized power—they have always generated performative and symbolic effects in excess of their obdurately material ones. They have produced and negated certain political imaginaries. They have contributed to the political subjectivity of those they encompass and those they exclude. Medieval walls and fortresses dotting the European countryside, for example, officially built against invasion, also served to overawe and hence bind and pacify the towns they encircled. More generally, all walls defining or defending political entities have shaped collective and individual identity within as they aimed to block penetration from without" (ibid., 40).

53. Amy Chazkel and David Serlin, "Editors' Introduction," *Radical History Review*, no. 108 (Fall 2010): 1–10.

54. "However architecturally interesting or complex, walls are conventionally regarded as functional instruments for dividing, separating, retaining, protecting, shoring up, or supporting. Whether constructing a building, holding back land erosion, or limning neighbourhoods, walls are ordinarily perceived as intended for a material task. Yet walls are also commonly said to convey moods or feelings by their design, placement, and relationship to built or natural environments. They may set or foreclose political and economic possibilities and be screens for a host of projected desires, needs, or anxieties" (Brown, *Walled States*, 73).

55. Ibid., 74.

56. Ibid., 76.

57. Ibid., 24.

58. Ibid., 22.

59. "In the discourse of civilizational struggle that has superseded Cold War discourse in organizing the global imaginary of liberal democracies, two disparate images are merged to produce a single figure of danger justifying exclusion and closure: the hungry masses, on the one hand, and cultural-religious aggression toward Western values, on the other" (ibid., 33).

60. Ibid., 25.

61. Ibid., 69.

62. Lissak, *Mass Immigration*, 62.

63. Brown, *Walled States*, 108.

64. Ibid., 107.

65. Ibid.

66. Ibid., 26.

67. Ibid., 81. This also echoes back to Mary Douglas: "We have seen that powers are attributed to any structure of ideas and that rules of avoidance make a visible public recognition of its boundaries" (*Purity and Danger*, 188).

68. Brown, *Walled States*, 26.

69. Robert Frost, "Mending Wall," Academy of American Poets, accessed September 9, 2014, https://www.poets.org/poetsorg/poem/mending-wall.

70. Ibid.

71. Some examples of Brown's take on theatricality are as follows: "If walls do not actually accomplish the interdiction fueling and legitimating them, if they perversely institutionalize the contested and degraded status of the boundaries they limn, they nevertheless stage both sovereign jurisdiction and an aura of sovereign power and awe" (*Walled State*, 26). She continues, "They also resurrect an image of the state as sustaining the very powers of protection and self-determination

challenged by terrorist technologies, on one side, and neoliberal capitalism, on the other. They are potential spectacles of such protection and self-determination and more generally of the resolve and capacity for action identified with the political autonomy generated by sovereignty" (92).

72. Michel Foucault, *Discipline and Punish: The Birth of the Prison* (New York: Vintage Books, 1995), 197.

73. Ibid., 199.

74. Ibid., 208.

75. Douglas, *Purity and Danger*, 15.

76. Ann Dally, "The Development of Western Medical Science," in *Medicine: A History of Healing*, ed. Roy Porter (New York: Marlowe, 1997), 66.

77. Ibid., 67.

78. Roy Porter, *The Greatest Benefit to Mankind: A Medical History of Humanity* (New York: W. W. Norton, 1997).

79. Dally, "The Development of Western Medical Science," 63.

80. For more on twentieth-century medicine and power, see Porter, *Greatest Benefit to Mankind*; Jacalyn Duffin, *History of Medicine: A Scandalously Short Introduction* (Toronto: University of Toronto Press, 1999); Allan Brandt, *The Cigarette Century: The Rise, Fall, and Deadly Persistence of the Product That Defined America* (New York: Basic Books, 2009); Paul Farmer, *Infections and Inequalities: The Modern Plagues* (Berkeley: University of California Press, 2001); Rebecca Skloot, *The Immortal Life of Henrietta Lacks* (New York: Broadway Books, 2011).

81. "For a golden moment in the mid-1960's it was possible to imagine that infectious diseases might some day be eradicated completely" (Patrice Bourdelais, *Epidemics Laid Low: A History of What Happened in Rich Countries* [Baltimore: Johns Hopkins University Press, 2006], 128).

82. The Doctors' Trial at Nuremberg (1946–1947) was a watershed event that cast a shadow on the moral authority of European medical science and medical practitioners. The public trial of leading physicians and medical researchers raised questions that eventually created a growing awareness of the atrocities committed in the name of medicine—which we see in the drafting of the Nuremberg Code and eugenics' fall from grace. These helped mark an era in which declarations of human rights were beginning to permeate the world of medicine, as well as the perception of medical authority, and redefine accepted notions of medical power, the rights of the sick and weak, and boundaries of state power. The late 1940s and 1950s was a period in which the authority and standing of Western medicine was still largely intact but in which the wheels of change were beginning to turn—even if only just barely beginning. On the Nuremberg Doctors' Trial, the Nuremberg Code, and their impact on biomedicine, see Paul Weindling, "The

Origins of Informed Consent: The International Scientific Commission on Medical War Crimes, and the Nuremberg Code," *Bulletin of the History of Medicine* 75, no. 1 (2001): 37–71.

83. See, for example, Roy Porter's description of compulsory vaccinations and examinations in the nineteenth century, Porter, *Greatest Benefit to Mankind*, 128–140. As Warwick Anderson reminds us, "It is often forgotten that in the name of public health the state is licensed to palpate, handle, bruise, test and mobilize individuals, especially those deemed dangerous or marginal or needy" (Warwick Anderson, *Colonial Pathologies: American Tropical Medicine, Race, and Hygiene in the Philippines* [Durham: Duke University Press, 2006], 161).

84. Sandra M. Sufian, *Healing the Land and the Nation: Malaria and the Zionist Project in Palestine, 1920–1947* (Chicago: University of Chicago Press, 2007); Dafna Hirsch, "'Interpreters of the Occident to the Awakening Orient': The Jewish Public Health Nurse in Mandate Palestine," *Comparative Studies in Society and History* 50, no. 1 (2008): 227–255; Nadav Davidovitch and Rhona Seidelman, "Herzl's Altneuland: Zionist Utopia, Medical Science and Public Health," *Korot: The Israel Journal of the History of Medicine and Science*, 17 (2003–2004): 1–21.

85. Douglas, *Purity and Danger*, 85.

86. CZA, AK 456/3, Letter from Mapai Cell in *Shaar Ha'aliya* to Mapai Office, Tel Aviv, 23.3.51. An acronym for "Israel Workers' Party," Mapai was the dominant political party in Israel's early years.

87. S. Ilan Troen, *Imagining Zion: Dreams, Designs, and Realities in a Century of Jewish Settlement* (New Haven, Conn.: Yale University Press, 2003), 195, 205.

88. Much of this report's persuasiveness comes from the fact that it does not whitewash or simplify the descriptions of camp life, nor does it overly heroicize the staff. While it praises their efforts it does not glorify their practices; it is relatively open about their own shortcomings. The narratives of both the members of Mapai and the director alike are an expression of their frustration—first of all with these circumstances, but then, even more so, with the Yishuv. The sense is that by making Shaar Ha'aliya such an accepted target for criticism, the Yishuv was, in fact, making the staff's work harder and perhaps making scapegoats out of the people actually trying to do something while the bigger problems (i.e., clashes between the immigrants' expectations and Israeli absorption policy and nation building) were ultimately beyond their control.

89. CZA, AK 456/3, Letter from Mapai Cell in Shaar H'aaliya to Mapai Office, Tel Aviv, 23.3.51.

90. In *Israel: A History*, Anita Shapira gives a useful explanation of the weekly newspaper *Ha'olam Hazeh*, its political and cultural role and its editor Uri Avneri. Anita Shapira, *Israel: A History* (Waltham, Mass.: Brandeis University Press, 2014), 201.

91. Refael Sela, "Shaar Le *Aliya* oh Mahaneh Hesger?" [A gate for *Aliya* or a quarantine?], *Haolam Hazeh*, March 31, 1951.

92. On Nordau, Zionism, and the concept of degeneration, see George L. Mosse, "Max Nordau, Liberalism and the New Jew," *Journal of Contemporary History* 27, no. 4 (October 1992); Meira Weiss, *The Chosen Body* (Stanford: Stanford University Press, 2002).

93. CZA, AK 456/6, "Shaara Shel Yisrael" [Israel's Gate] by Pinchas Yorman.

94. I am convinced that this photo was taken at an earlier date, perhaps before Shaar Ha'aliya opened in 1949. In 1951, it would be practically impossible for the camp to be so empty. Even at the crack of dawn, people would already have been standing in crowded lines.

95. Strange and Bashford, *Isolation*, 15.

96. Douglas, *Purity and Danger*, 192.

97. Strange and Bashford, *Isolation*, 4.

CHAPTER 4 — MEMORY

1. For some of the major historiographical works that mention Shaar Ha'aliya, see Dvora Hacohen, *Immigrants in Turmoil: The Great Wave of Immigration to Israel and Its Absorption, 1948–1953* [in Hebrew] (Jerusalem: Yad Yitzhak Ben Tzvi, 1994); Orit Bashkin, *Impossible Exodus: Iraqi Jews in Israel* (Stanford: Stanford University Press, 2017); Orit Rozin, *The Rise of the Individual in 1950s Israel: A Challenge to Collectivism* (Waltham, Mass.: Brandeis University Press, 2011); S. Ilan Troen, *Imagining Zion: Dreams, Designs, and Realities in a Century of Jewish Settlement* (New Haven, Conn.: Yale University Press, 2003).

2. Yosef Hayim Yerushalmi, *Zakhor: Jewish History and Jewish Memory* (New York: Schocken Books, 1982), 109.

3. For the distinctions between memory and remembrance as well as categorization of historical remembrances, see Jay Winter, *Remembering War: The Great War between Memory and History in the Twentieth Century* (New Haven, Conn.: Yale University Press, 2006), 276.

4. On Israeli mythology, see Yael Zerubavel, *Recovered Roots: Collective Memory and the Making of Israeli National Tradition* (Chicago: University of Chicago Press, 1995); David Ohana, *The Origins of Israeli Mythology* (Cambridge: Cambridge University Press, 2012); Michael Feige and David Ohana, "Funeral at the Edge of a Cliff: Israel Bids Farewell to David Ben-Gurion," *Journal of Israeli History* 31, no. 2 (2012): 249–281.

5. Mordecai Naor, *The Atlit Camp: A Story of a Time and Place* (Israel: Atlit Heritage Site, 2010), 5.

6. Tamar Katriel explains that in this way the visitors are "invited to identify with the heroic struggle associated with the survivor's arrival in the Land of Israel (and, by extension, the new life they sought to build there)" (Tamar Katriel, "From Shore to Shore: The Holocaust, Clandestine, Immigration, and Israeli Heritage Museums," in *Visual Culture and the Holocaust*, ed. Barbie Zelizer [New Jersey: Rutgers University Press, 2001], 209).

7. Ibid., 6.

8. The top image on the heritage site's official pamphlet is a photograph of the camp from behind a barbed wire fence. *The Atlit "Illegal" Immigrant Detention Camp*, official heritage site pamphlet (2012). The top two of three photographs on the booklet by Mordecai Naor, *Atlit Camp*, show people in the camp detained behind barbed wire.

9. A sign on the disinfection hut in the Atlit Heritage Museum reads "When [disinfection] was completed, detainees were transferred to residential huts and held behind barbed wire fences. For survivors of the Holocaust, this 'reception' was a fresh reminder of the horrors of the German concentration camps."

10. Naor, *Atlit Camp*, 5, 38, 40, 42, 43, 45, 46, 61, 65, 75.

11. Ibid., 38.

12. Ibid., 42.

13. Ibid., 43.

14. Ibid., 65.

15. Zehavit Rotenberg, "The Atlit Detention Camp," in Naor, *Atlit Camp*, 5.

16. Naor, *Atlit Camp*, 55. A few pages later, in the testimony of the Palmach commander who led the raid, there is another brief reference to these men: "In the instructions that I had received regarding the breakout, I was told that three prisoners were suspected of having cooperated with the Nazis and would be left behind in the camp" (64).

17. Ibid., 5.

18. On Shaar Ha'aliya Bet, see Central Zionist Archive (CZA), AK 456/3, Untitled document written after 1954, and CZA, AK 456/1, "Distribution of the Aliya from Ports of Arrival, 1.4.51–12.8.54." While one document suggests that twenty-two thousand people went through Shaar Ha'aliya Bet (CZA, AK 456/3, Untitled Document from Weisberger's Files, Written after 1954), another document claims that the figure was actually forty-two thousand (CZA, AK 456/1, "Distribution of the *Aliya* from Ports of Arrival," 1.4.51–12.8.54).

19. Pierre Nora, *Rethinking France. Les Lieux de Mémoire*, vol. 1 (Chicago: University of Chicago Press, 2001), vii.

20. Ibid.

21. Ibid., xv.

22. Katriel, "From Shore to Shore," 209. For the development of Katriel's framework of study on Israeli museums and remembrance, see Tamar Katriel, *Performing the Past: A Study of Israel Settlement Museums* (London: Routledge, 1997).

23. Winter, *Remembering War*, 24.

24. Yerushalmi, *Zakhor*, 113.

25. Nora, *Rethinking France*, xi–xii.

26. Winter, *Remembering War*, 105.

27. Victoria Freeman, "'Toronto Has No History!' Indigeneity, Settler Colonialism, and Historical Memory in Canada's Largest City,'" *Urban History Review / Revue d'historie urbaine* 38, no. 2 (Spring 2010): 21–35.

28. Yerushalmi, *Zakhor*, 113.

29. Freeman, "'Toronto Has No History!,'" 22. On the construction of memory, see Alan Gordon, *Making Public Pasts: The Contested Terrain of Montreal's Public Memories, 1891–1930* (Montreal: McGill-Queen's University Press, 2001); Barry Schwartz, *Abraham Lincoln in the Post-Heroic Era* (Chicago: University of Chicago Press, 2008); Barry Schwartz, *Abraham Lincoln and the Forge of National Memory* (Chicago: University of Chicago Press, 2000).

30. Katriel, "'From Shore to Shore,'" 209.

31. Ibid.

32. Zerubavel, *Recovered Roots*, xviii.

33. Hanna Yablonka, "The Development of Holocaust Consciousness in Israel: The Nuremberg, Kapos, Kastner, and Eichmann Trials," *Israel Studies* 8, no. 3 (Fall 2003): 1–24.

34. Hanna Yablonka, *Survivors of the Holocaust* (London: Macmillan, 1999).

35. Winter, *Remembering War*, 277.

36. Ibid., 9.

37. Eli Amir, *Tarnegol kaparot* [*Scapegoat*] (Tel Aviv: Am Oved, 1990), 1.

38. Eli Amir, *Maphriah Hayonim* [The Dove Flyer] (Tel Aviv: Am Oved, 1992), 414.

39. Ibid., 419.

40. Ibid., 423–424.

41. Eli Amir, "The Rooster Still Reads," interview, *Ynet*, April 16, 2010, http://www.ynet.co.il/articles/0,7340,L-3873104,00.html.

42. "Eliamir.com" (entry on Eli Amir) [in Hebrew], *Simania*, accessed November 8, 2013, http://simania.co.il/authorDetails.php?itemId=4953.

43. Chava Alberstein, "Hamehagrim," 1986.

44. *The Jewish Women's Archive*, s.v. "Chava Alberstein," accessed November 8, 2013, http://jwa.org/encyclopedia/article/alberstein-chava; Simon Broughton, "The Joan Baez of Israel," *Jewish Quarterly* 43, no. 4 (1996): 55–56.

45. The line "Nothing was as promised" is followed by "They promised a warm land / there were winds and storms." But the anonymous "they" making these promises is left to our imagination. Certainly, this could be understood as Jewish Agency representatives. But that "they" could just as easily be friends and family members who had immigrated earlier and who whitewashed their own stories. The only explicit reference to any state agents is the line "מרכז הסברה מביא סרטים וכיסאות" (The PR department brings movies and chairs)—which is an innocuous image.

46. David Belahsan and Asher Nehemias, *The Ringworm Children* (Israel: 2003).

47. Baruch Modan et al., "Radiation-Induced Head and Neck Tumors," *Lancet* 303, no. 7852 (February 23, 1974): 277–279. For the history of Shaar Ha'aliya's Ringworm and Trachoma Institute, see Rhona Seidelman, S. Ilan Troen, and Shifra Shvarts, "'Healing' the Bodies and Souls of Immigrant Children: The Ringworm and Trachoma Institute, Shaar Ha'aliya, Israel 1952–1960," *Journal of Israeli History* 29, no. 2 (2010): 191–211.

48. For further reading on the compensation law, see Nadav Davidovitch and Avital Margalit, "Public Health, Law, and Traumatic Collective Experiences: The Case of Mass Ringworm Irradiations," in *Trauma and Memory: Reading, Healing and Making Law*, ed. Austin Sarat, Nadav Davidovitch, and Michal Alberstein (Stanford: Stanford University Press, 2008).

49. One channel that has the entire movie has had almost three thousand views. *The Ringworm Children testing of large radiation doses on humans*, YouTube video, 44:41, posted by vidsupquick on September 8, 2011, http://www.youtube.com/watch?v=vMp1tef4lg4, accessed December 7, 2012.

50. I am using the English subtitles, translated from the Hebrew, that appear in the film.

51. On the *konseptziya*, see Benny Morris, *Righteous Victims: A History of the Zionist-Arab Conflict 1881–2001* (New York: Vintage Books, 2001), 443; Agranat Commission, "Interim Report," *Israel in the Middle East: Documents and Readings on Society, Politics and Foreign Relations, Pre-1948 to the Present*, ed. Itamar Rabinovich and Jehuda Reinharz, 2nd ed. (Waltham, Mass.: Brandeis University Press, 2008), 278–284.

52. Comments made by David Belahsan in *Panim Amitiot Im Amnon Levi*. "*Panim Amitiot: Sodot Hagazezet*," online video, broadcast November 4, 2018.

53. Seidelman, Troen, and Shvarts, "'Healing' the Bodies and Souls," 197.

54. Frédéric Charbonneau, "Quarantine and Caress," in *Imagining Contagion in Early Modern Europe*, ed. Claire L. Carlin (Basingstoke, U.K.: Palgrave Macmillan, 2005).

55. This was a comment by Dr. Dana Blander following a panel at the Israel Studies Association in UCLA, 2013.

56. For some of the challenges and discrimination that Holocaust survivors faced upon their arrival in Israel, see Yablonka, *Survivors of the Holocaust*; Yablonka, "Development of Holocaust Consciousness"; Tom Segev, *The Seventh Million*. On perceptions of the ideal, healthy Israeli body, see Meira Weiss, *The Chosen Body* (Stanford: Stanford University Press, 2002); *Korot: The Israel Journal of the History of Medicine and Science* 17 (2003–2004): 1–21; Rozin, *Rise of the Individual*.

57. Aharon Appelfeld, *A Table for One: Under the Light of Jerusalem* (London: Toby, 2007), 15–16.

58. Like so many successful, mainstream Israeli musicians, Alberstein began her career during her military service when she served as part of the military band. For more on the Israeli army band and the various routes into the Israeli music scene, see Motti Regev and Edwin Seroussi, *Popular Music and National Culture in Israel* (Berkeley: University of California Press, 2004).

59. Eli Amir, *On Writing*, YouTube video, 13:07, posted by Willem Sternberg on June 16, 2012, http://www.youtube.com/watch?v=sNVPCmLcb9Y&feature=youtu.be.

60. Shlomo Bar and the Brera Hativit, *Metoch Kelim Shvurim*, 1985. (See "Discography," accessed November 16, 2013, http://www.shlomobar.com).

61. CZA, AK 456/6, Notes from December 28, 1955 for a Presentation on Shaar Ha'aliya at the Twenty-Fourth Zionist Congress.

62. CZA, AK 456/2, Weisberger Letter, 3.9.52.

63. Seidelman, Troen, and Shvarts, "The Press and the War against Ringworm," in "'Healing' the Bodies and Souls of Immigrant Children," 201–204.

64. "Holei gazezet ve-hagarenet mitrapim be-Shaar Ha'aliya" [People ill with ringworm and trachoma heal at Sha'ar ha-Aliyah], *Davar*, May 20, 1955.

65. "Ra'iti shamati: 'Shaar Ha'aliya'—machine ripui" [I saw and heard: Shaar Ha'aliya—healing camp], *Ha'aretz*, May 29, 1955.

66. Theodor Herzl, *Altneuland: Old-New Land*, trans. Paula Arnold (Haifa, Israel: Haifa, 1960), 87. See also Steven Beller, *Herzl* (New York: Grove Weindenfeld, 1991), 87.

67. David F. Musto, "Quarantine and the Problem of AIDS," *Milbank Quarterly* 64, supp. 1 (1986): 104.

68. David Deri, dir., *The Ancestral Sin* (Israel: D. D. Productions, 2017).

69. Sasson Somekh, *Call It Dreaming: Memoirs 1951–2000* [in Hebrew] (Israel: Hakibbutz Hamehuad, Sifrei Siman Kriya, 2008), 15.

70. Avraham Harman Institute of Contemporary Jewry, Oral History Division (hereafter OHD), (210), 136, 12.

71. OHD, (210), 138; OHD, (210), 142; OHD, (210), 136.

72. OHD, (210), 138; OHD, (210), 163; OHD, (210), 136.

73. OHD, (210), 158; Rhona Seidelman interview with S. H., 23.10.05. This interview was conducted as part of a research project directed by Prof. Shifra Shvarts, the Israel Science Foundation, 1217/04.

74. Rhona Seidelman interview with V. S. 21.11.05, Beer Sheva, Israel. This interview was conducted as part of a research project directed by Prof. Shifra Shvarts, the Israel Science Foundation, 1217/04.

75. Rhona Seidelman interview with E. S. 27.09.05, Beer Sheva, Israel. This interview was conducted as part of a research project directed by Prof. Shifra Shvarts, the Israel Science Foundation, 1217/04.

76. OHD, (210), 113, 13.

77. OHD, (210), 113, 34.

78. On the Shaar Ha'aliya administration's perception of Iraqi immigrants as troublemakers, see "Behitarvut hamishtara yatzu keh-2000 *olim* le ma'abarot" [2,000 *Olim* left for *Ma'abarot* with police intervention], *Maariv*, August 8, 1951.

79. OHD, (210), 19.

80. OHD, (210), 122, 4.

81. OHD, (210), 112, 6.

82. Charbonneau, "Quarantine and Caress," 124.

83. OHD, (210), 141, Sylvia Meltzer Interview, 1993.

84. OHD, (210), 138.

85. His words were מחנה מעבר.

86. OHD, (210), 138, Interview with Yaacov Steiner.

87. OHD, (210), 136.

88. From a 1977 quote in the book's introduction, one gets a sense of the urgency Yehuda felt about his calling: "And yet another mission is before me; to finally write the book on 'Shaar Ha'aliya'. All the people who worked in absorption of the *Aliya* after the establishment of the State are disappearing one by one . . . I have been left to tell the story of the Ingathering of the Exiles. I have decided to take all the material with me [to India] and sit down and write—and write" (Yehuda Weisberger, *Shaar Ha'aliya: The Diary of the Mass Aliya, 1947–1957* [in Hebrew] [Jerusalem: Bialik Institute, 1985], 7).

89. See, for example, Anita Shapira's chapter on the mass immigration in her 2014 book *Israel: A History* (Waltham, Mass.: Brandeis University Press, 2014); the references Orit Rozin makes to Shaar Ha'aliya in her works on the mass immigration, both in *Rise of the Individual* as well as in her later book *A Home for All Jews: Citizenship, Rights, and National Identity in the New Israeli State* (Waltham, Mass.: Brandeis University Press, 2016); Nadav Davidovitch and Shifra Shvarts, "Health and Hegemony: Preventive Medicine, Immigration and the Israeli Melting Pot," *Israel Studies* 9, no. 2 (2004): 150–179.

90. In 1949, he was chosen by the Jewish Agency to be the first director of *Shaar Ha'aliya*. At that time, he had been working as the head of the immigrant absorption center Neve Haim, located near Hadera. Although he officially left his position as *Shaar Ha'aliya* director only in May 1957, he had been on a leave of absence since 1956 while doing immigration work in Tunis (see CZA, AK 456/1, Administrative Report #81, 14.2.56; CZA, AK 456/2, Letter of Recommendation for Weisberger from Jewish Agency, Outlining Details of His Work from 1947 to 1960, 1.1.60). After leaving *Shaar Ha'aliya*, he continued his work in absorption in the position of "district supervisor in the Division for the Absorption of Professionals and *Olim* from Western Countries" (see CZA, AK 456/2, Letter of Recommendation for Weisberger from Jewish Agency, 1.1.60).

91. Weisberger, *Shaar Ha'aliya*, 63.

92. His remarks often generalize about ethnic groups but do not fall into a simplistic Ashkenazi/Sephardic dichotomy. He is critical of Romanians but not Bulgarians. His description of "Bnei Yisrael" immigrants from India is very derogatory (ibid., 103). He says of Iraqi immigrants that it is a "pity they go bad quickly" (101).

93. Ibid., 71.

94. Ibid. I have translated בתי עולים as immigrant centers.

95. With this in mind, the limited reference to the barbed wire fence, and the absence of any mention of quarantine, are well suited to the place that these subjects have held in Israeli discourse, as discussed in the introduction.

96. Avraham Sternberg, *A People Is Absorbed* (Tel Aviv: Hakibbutz Hameuhad, 1973), 126.

97. Ibid., 22.

98. Ibid., 156.

99. Ibid., 124.

100. Ibid., 125.

101. Yerushalmi, *Zakhor*, 109.

CONCLUSION

1. I turn again to Strange and Bashford: "The inseparability and the recurrent intertwining of 'prevention,' 'punishment' and 'protection' reveals the historic connection between all these state-endorsed practices in modernity, as well as between the populations rendered into 'problems'" (Carolyn Strange and Alison Bashford, eds., *Isolation: Places and Practices of Exclusion* [London: Routledge, 2003], 222).

2. Amnon Rubenstein, "The Israeli Left. 1970," in *Israel in the Middle East: Documents and Readings on Society, Politics and Foreign Relations, Pre-1948 to the Present*, ed. Itamar Rabinovich and Jehuda Reinharz, 2nd ed. (Waltham, Mass.: Brandeis University Press, 2008), 227.

3. CZA, AK 456/1, Letter from Kalman Levin to Dr. Berman, 14.3.51.

EPILOGUE

1. Tony Judt, *The Memory Chalet* (London: Penguin, 2010), 162.

2. A partial model for this memorial would be the Museum of the History of Medicine in the Faculty of Health Sciences, Ben-Gurion University of the Negev. This museum relies on beautiful, enlarged historical photographs.

3. In Hebrew it would be מוזיאון שער העלייה להגירה ורפואה, "Muzeon Shaar Ha'aliya Le Hagira Ve Refuah."

4. CZA, AK 456/6, "Shaara Shel Yisrael," by Pinchas Yorman.

5. A Hebrew transcript of Yishai's comments can be found at http://www.ynet.co.il/ articles/0,7340,L-3798115,00.html. A video of his full interview on "Pgosh et ha itonut" (Meet the press) can be found in the program's archives, http://www.reshet.ynet.co .il. Numerous responses to these comments came out in the media. For a few of the responses, see Yossi Sarid, "Virusim" [Viruses], *Haaretz*, November 6, 2009. Rhona Seidelman, "Al mehagrim ve mahalot" [Immigrants, Disease and the Zionist Ethos], *Haaretz*, November 11, 2009. "Oy le ota busha" [Oh, to the same shame], editorial, *Haaretz*, November 5, 2009. The talkbacks to each of the articles and videos give an indication of the broad range of issues and opinions that the comments evoked.

6. Rhona Seidelman, "Al mehagrim ve mahalot" [Immigrants, Disease and the Zionist Ethos], *Haaretz*, November 11, 2009.

7. See Don Seeman, *One People, One Blood: Ethiopian-Israelis and the Return to Judaism* (New Brunswick, N.J.: Rutgers University Press, 2010).

8. Talia Nesher, "Israel Admits Ethiopian Women Were Given Birth Control Shots," *Haaretz*, January 7, 2013, http://www.haaretz.com/news/national/israel -admits-ethiopian-women-were-given-birth-control-shots.premium-1.496519; Talia Nesher, "Why Is the Birth Rate in Israel's Ethiopian Community Declining?," *Haaretz*, December 9, 2012, http://www.haaretz.com/news/national/why-is-the -birth-rate-in-israel-s-ethiopian-community-declining.premium-1.483494.

9. For further reading on the compensation law, see Nadav Davidovitch and Avital Margalit, "Public Health, Law, and Traumatic Collective Experiences: The Case of Mass Ringworm Irradiations," in *Trauma and Memory: Reading, Healing and Making Law*, ed. Austin Sarat, Nadav Davidovitch, and Michal Alberstein

(Stanford: Stanford University Press, 2008); Eyal Katvan, "Picking the Sores of the Past: Physical, Mental and Medical Examinations under the Compensation of Ringworm Law (1994)" (paper presented at annual conference, Association of Israel Studies, Beer Sheva, Israel, June 2009).

10. H. Markel and A. M. Stern, "The Foreignness of Germs: The Persistent Association of Immigrants and Disease in American Society," *Milbank Quarterly* 80, no. 4 (2002): 757–788.

11. Refael Sela, "Shaar Le *Aliya* oh Mahaneh Hesger?" [A gate for *Aliya* or a quarantine?], *Haolam Hazeh*, March 31, 1951.

12. Here I am paraphrasing a statement made by a woman shown in the movie *The Ringworm Children*.

13. David Biale, *Power and Powerlessness in Jewish History* (New York: Schocken Books, 1986), 9.

Bibliography

Allen, Shannen K., and Richard D. Semba. "The Trachoma 'Menace' in the United States, 1897–1960." *History of Ophthalmology* 47, no. 5 (September–October 2002): 500–509.

Alroey, Gur. "Exiles in Their Country? The Story of the Tel-Aviv and Jaffa Refugees in the Lower Galilee, 1917–1918" [in Hebrew]. *Catedra* 120 (2010): 135–160.

———. *An Unpromising Land: Jewish Migration to Palestine in the Early Twentieth Century.* Stanford: Stanford University Press, 2014.

Amir, Eli. *Maphriah Hayonim.* Tel Aviv: Am Oved, 1992.

———. *Tarnegol kaparot* [*Scapegoat*]. Tel Aviv: Am Oved, 1990.

Anderson, Warwick. *Colonial Pathologies: American Tropical Medicine, Race, and Hygiene in the Philippines.* Durham, N.C.: Duke University Press, 2006.

Annas, George J., and Michael A. Grodin. *The Nazi Doctors and the Nuremberg Code: Human Rights in Human Experimentation.* New York: Oxford University Press, 1992.

Appelfeld, Aharon. *A Table for One: Under the Light of Jerusalem.* London: Toby, 2007.

Arnon, Yishay. "Mediniut haaliya ve klita ba shanim 1954–56: Yesuma ve totzootea" [Aliya and absorption policy 1954–56: Application and results]. In *Kibbutz galuyot: Ha-aliyah le-Eretz Yisrael, mitos u-metzi'ut* [Ingathering of exiles: Aliyah to the land of Israel, myth, and reality], edited by Dvora Hacochen, 317–341. Jerusalem: Zalman Shazar Center for Jewish History, 1998.

The Atlit "Illegal" Immigrant Detention Camp. Official heritage site pamphlet, 2012.

Auerbach, Jerold S. *Brothers at War: Israel and the Tragedy of the Altalena.* New Orleans: Quid Pro Books, 2011.

Avineri, Shlomo. *The Making of Modern Zionism: The Intellectual Origins of the Jewish State*. New York: Basic Books, 1981.

Bar-El, Dan. "Cholera Epidemics in Palestine, 1865–1918" [in Hebrew]. PhD diss., Bar-Ilan University, 2006.

———. *Ruah ra'ah: Magefot ha-kholerah ve-hitpathut ha-refu'ah be-Eretz-Yisrael beshalhei ha-tkufah ha-otmanit* [An ill wind: Cholera epidemics and medical development in Palestine in the late Ottoman period]. Jerusalem: Bialik Institute, 2010.

Barell, Ari. *Engineer King: David Ben-Gurion, Science and Nation Building* [in Hebrew]. Sde Boker, Israel: Sde Boker Research Institute for the Study of Israel and Zionism, 2014.

———. "Ha manheeg, ha madanim ve ha milchama: David Ben-Gurion ve hakamat heyil ha mada" [Leader, Scientists and War: David Ben-Gurion and the Establishment of the Science Corps]. *Yisrael* 15 (2009): 67–92.

———. "Leviathan ve ha academia: haim haya nisayon lehaalim et ha universita ha ivrit beshnoteyha a rishonot shel midinat yisrael?" [Leviathan and Academia: Was There an Attempt to Nationalize the Hebrew University in the Early Years of the State of Israel?] *Tarbut Democratit* 13 (2011): 7–59.

Bashan, Rafael. "Kol Adam Hamishi Baaretz Yashav Kahn" [Every fifth person in the country sat here]. *Ma'ariv*, February 9, 1962.

Bashkin, Orit. *Impossible Exodus: Iraqi Jews in Israel*. Stanford: Stanford University Press, 2017.

Batelli, Clement F. "Youth Interest High in War against Tuberculosis." *Health* 73, no. 6 (June 1946).

Beller, Steven. *Herzl*. New York: Grove Weindenfeld, 1991.

Biale, David. *Power and Powerlessness in Jewish History*. New York: Schocken Books, 1986.

Bilmus, Birsen. *Plague, Quarantine and Geopolitics in the Ottoman Empire*. Edinburgh: Edinburgh University Press, 2011.

Bossuat, Gerard. "French Development and Co-operation under de Gaulle." *Contemporary European History* 12, no. 4 (November 2003): 432–436.

Bourdelais, Patrice. *Epidemics Laid Low: A History of What Happened in Rich Countries*. Baltimore: Johns Hopkins University Press, 2006.

Brandt, Allan. *The Cigarette Century: The Rise, Fall, and Deadly Persistence of the Product That Defined America*. New York: Basic Books, 2009.

Broughton, Simon. "The Joan Baez of Israel." *Jewish Quarterly* 43, no. 4 (1996): 55–56.

Brown, Wendy. *Walled States, Waning Sovereignty*. New York: Zone Books, 2010.

Carmi, Boris. *Photographs from Israel*. Edited by Alexandra Nocke. Munich: Prestel, 2004.

Cartier, Raymond. "Israël: Étendue: Trois départements Mission: Résoudre dans le monde le problème juif." *Paris-Match*, August 13, 1949.

Charbonneau, Frédéric. "Quarantine and Caress." In *Imagining Contagion in Early Modern Europe*, edited by Claire L. Carlin. Basingstoke, U.K.: Palgrave Macmillan, 2005.

Chazkel, Amy, and David Serlin. "Editors' Introduction." *Radical History Review* 2010, no. 108 (Fall 2010): 1–10.

Dahan-Kalev, Henrietta. "Israeli Identity—between New Immigrants and 'Oldtimers.'" In *Israel in the Great Wave of Immigration, 1948–1953* [in Hebrew], edited by Dalia Ofer. Jerusalem: Yad Yitzhak Ben Tzvi, 1996.

———. "You're So Pretty—You Don't Look Moroccan." *Israel Studies* 6, no. 1 (2001): 1–13.

Dally, Ann. "The Development of Western Medical Science." In *Medicine: A History of Healing*, edited by Roy Porter. New York: Marlowe, 1997.

Davidovitch, Nadav, and Avital Margalit. "Public Health, Law, and Traumatic Collective Experiences: The Case of Mass Ringworm Irradiations." In *Trauma and Memory: Reading, Healing and Making Law*, edited by Austin Sarat, Nadav Davidovitch, and Michal Alberstein. Stanford: Stanford University Press, 2008.

Davidovitch, Nadav, and Rhona Seidelman. "Herzl's *Altneuland*: Zionist Utopia, Medical Science and Public Health." *Korot: The Israel Journal of the History of Medicine and Science* 17 (2003–2004): 1–21.

Davidovitch, Nadav, Rhona Seidelman, and Shifra Shvarts. "Contested Bodies: Medicine, Public Health and Mass Immigration to Israel." In *Reapproaching Borders: New Perspectives on the Study of Israel-Palestine*, edited by Sandy Suffian and Mark Levine. Lanham, Md.: Rowman & Littlefield, 2007.

Davidovitch, Nadav, and Shifra Shvarts. "Health and Hegemony: Preventive Medicine, Immigration and the Israeli Melting Pot." *Israel Studies* 9, no. 2 (2004): 150–179.

Davies, Michael A. "Health and Disease in Israel, 1948–1994." In *Health and Disease in the Holy Land: Studies in the History and Sociology of Medicine from Ancient Times to the Present*, edited by Manfred Waserman and Samuel S. Kottek. Lewiston, N.Y.: Edwin Mellen, 1996.

Diamond, James A. "Maimonides on Leprosy: Illness as Contemplative Metaphor." *Jewish Quarterly Review* 96, no. 1 (Winter 2006): 95–122.

Ding, Huiling. "Transnational Quarantine Rhetoric: Mandatory, Voluntary, and Coerced Quarantines, Public Communication, and Stigmatization in SARS and H1N1 Flu." *Journal of Medical Humanities* 35 (2014): 191–210.

Dols, Michael W. "The Leper in Islamic Society." *Speculum* 58, no. 4 (1983): 891–916.

Douglas, Mary. *Purity and Danger: An Analysis of Pollution and Taboo*. London: Penguin Books, 1970.

Duffin, Jacalyn. *History of Medicine: A Scandalously Short Introduction*. Toronto: University of Toronto Press, 1999.

Efron, John, Steven Weitzman, and Matthias Lehmann. *The Jews: A History*. 2nd ed. New York: Routledge, 2016.

"Eliamir.com" (entry on Eli Amir) [in Hebrew]. *Simania*. Accessed November 8, 2013. http://simania.co.il/authorDetails.php?itemId=4953.

Encyclopedia of the Black Death. Santa Barbara: ABC-CLIO, 2012.

Encyclopedia of the Founders and Builders of Israel. New York: Touro College Libraries, 2019. Accessed January 9, 2014. http://www.tidhar.tourolib.org/tidhar/view/15/4775.

Falk, Rafael. "The Settlement of Israel as a Eugenic Act" [in Hebrew]. *Alpayim* 23 (2002): 179–198.

Farmer, Paul. *Infections and Inequalities: The Modern Plagues*. Berkeley: University of California Press, 2001.

Feige, Michael, and David Ohana. "Funeral at the Edge of a Cliff: Israel Bids Farewell to David Ben-Gurion." *Journal of Israeli History* 31, no. 2 (2012): 249–281.

Foucault, Michel. *Discipline and Punish: The Birth of the Prison*. New York: Vintage Books, 1995.

Freeman, Victoria. "'Toronto Has No History!' Indigeneity, Settler Colonialism, and Historical Memory in Canada's Largest City." *Urban History Review / Revue d'historie urbaine* 38, no. 2 (Spring 2010): 21–35.

Garrett, Laurie. *The Coming Plague: Newly Emerging Diseases in a World Out of Balance*. New York: Penguin, 1994.

Glitzenstein, Esther Meir. *The "Magic Carpet" Exodus of Yemenite Jewry: An Israeli Formative Myth*. Sussex, U.K.: Sussex Academic, 2014.

———. *Zionism in an Arab Country: Jews in Iraq in the 1940s*. London: Routledge, 2004.

Goetz, Thomas. *The Remedy: Robert Koch, Arthur Conan Doyle and the Quest to Cure Tuberculosis*. New York: Gotham Books, 2014.

Gordon, Alan. *Making Public Pasts: The Contested Terrain of Montreal's Public Memories, 1891–1930*. Montreal: McGill-Queen's University Press, 2001.

Gross, Nachum. "Israel's Economy" [in Hebrew]. In *The First Decade* [in Hebrew], edited by Zvi Zameret and Hana Yablonka. Jerusalem: Yad Yitzhak Ben-Tzvi, 1997.

Grushka, Theodor. *Health Services in Israel*. Jerusalem: Ministry of Health, 1968.

Hacohen, Dvora. "From Fantasy to Reality—Ben-Gurion's Plan for Mass Immigration, 1942–1945." *Research Institute for the History of the Keren Kayemeth LeIsrael* [Jewish National Fund Land and Settlement] 18 (October 1995).

————. *Immigrants in Turmoil: The Great Wave of Immigration to Israel and Its Absorption, 1948–1953* [in Hebrew]. Jerusalem: Yad Yitzhak Ben Tzvi, 1994.

————, ed. *Kibbutz galuyot: Ha-aliyah le-Eretz Yisrael, mitos u-metzi'ut* [Ingathering of exiles: Aliyah to the land of Israel, myth, and reality]. Jerusalem: Zalman Shazar Center for Jewish History, 1998.

————. "Mediniyut ha-aliyah ba-asor ha-rishon la-medinah: Ha-nisyonot le-hagbalat ha-aliyah ve-goralam" [Immigration policy in the first decade of statehood: The attempts to restrict immigration and their outcome]. In *Kibbutz galuyot: Ha-aliyah le-Eretz Yisrael, mitos u-metzi'ut* [Ingathering of exiles: Aliyah to the land of Israel, myth, and reality], edited by Dvora Hacochen. Jerusalem: Zalman Shazar Center for Jewish History, 1998.

Halamish, Aviva. "Aliyah selektivit ba-ra'ayon, ba-ma'aseh uva-historiografiyah ha-tziyoniyim" [Selective immigration in Zionist ideology: Praxis and historiography]. In *Idan ha-tziyonut* [The age of Zionism], edited by Anita Shapira, Jehuda Reinharz, and Jay Harris, 185–202. Jerusalem: Zalman Shazar Center for Jewish History, 2000.

Harper, Kyle. *The Fate of Rome: Climate, Disease, and the End of an Empire.* Princeton: Princeton University Press, 2017.

Helman, Anat. *Becoming Israeli: National Ideals and Everyday Life in the 1950s.* Waltham, Mass.: Brandeis University Press, 2014.

Hertzberg, Arthur. *The Zionist Idea: A Historical Analysis and Reader.* Philadelphia: Jewish Publication Society, 1997.

Herzl, Theodor. *Altneuland: Old-New Land.* Translated by Paula Arnold. Haifa, Israel: Haifa, 1960.

Hirsch, Dafna. "'Interpreters of the Occident to the Awakening Orient': The Jewish Public Health Nurse in Mandate Palestine." *Comparative Studies in Society and History* 50, no. 1 (2008): 227–255.

————. *"We Are Here to Bring the West": Hygiene Education and Culture Building in the Jewish Society of Palestine during the British Mandate Period.* Sde Boker, Israel: Ben-Gurion Research Institute for the Study of Israel and Zionism, 2014.

Holtzman, Avner. "The Encounter between Newcomers and 'Oldtimers' as Reflected in Hebrew Fiction" [in Hebrew]. In *Israel in the Great Wave of Immigration, 1948–1953* [in Hebrew], edited by Dalia Ofer. Jerusalem: Yad Yitzhak Ben Tzvi, 1996.

Horowitz, Dan, and Moshe Lissak. *Trouble in Utopia: The Overburdened Polity of Israel.* Albany: State University of New York Press, 1989.

"In Memoriam: Ruth Gruber." *Holocaust and Genocide Studies* 31, no. 1 (Spring 2017): 185.

The Jewish Women's Archive. "Chava Alberstein." Accessed November 8, 2013. http://jwa.org/encyclopedia/article/alberstein-chava.

Judt, Tony. *The Memory Chalet.* London: Penguin, 2010.

Kahanoff, Jacqueline Shohet. *Mongrels or Marvels: The Levantine Writings of Jacqueline Shohet Kahanoff.* Edited by Deborah A. Starr and Sasson Somekh. Stanford: Stanford University Press, 2011.

Kark, Ruth. "Planning, Housing, and Land Policy 1948–1952: The Formation of Concepts of Governmental Frameworks." In *Israel: The First Decade of Independence,* edited by S. Ilan Troen and Noah Lucas, 461–495. Albany: State University of New York Press, 1995.

Katriel, Tamar. "From Shore to Shore: The Holocaust, Clandestine, Immigration, and Israeli Heritage Museums." In *Visual Culture and the Holocaust,* edited by Barbie Zelizer. New Brunswick, N.J.: Rutgers University Press, 2001.

———. *Performing the Past: A Study of Israel Settlement Museums.* London: Routledge, 1997.

Katvan, Eyal. "Picking the Sores of the Past: Physical, Mental and Medical Examinations under the Compensation of Ringworm Law (1994)." Paper presented at annual conference, Association of Israel Studies, Beer Sheva, Israel, June 2009.

Kelton, Paul. "Avoiding the Smallpox Spirits: Colonial Epidemics and Southeastern Indian Survival." *Ethnohistory* 51, no. 1 (Winter 2004): 45–71.

Kershaw, Alex. *Blood and Champagne: The Life and Times of Robert Capa.* London: Macmillan, 2002.

Khazzoom, Aziza. "Did the Israeli State Engineer Segregation? On the Placement of Jewish Immigrants in Development Towns in the 1950s." *Social Forces* 84, no. 1 (September 2005): 115–134.

Kiple, Kenneth F., ed. *The Cambridge World History of Human Disease.* Cambridge: Cambridge University Press, 1993.

Kirsh, Nurit. "The Beginning of Genetics in the Hebrew University." In *The History of the Hebrew University of Jerusalem* [in Hebrew], edited by Hagit Lavsky, vol. 2, 161–185. Jerusalem: Magnes, 2009.

———. "Genetic Research on Israel's Populations: Two Opposite Tendencies." In *Twentieth Century Ethics of Human Subjects Research: Historical Perspectives on Values, Practices, and Regulations,* edited by Volker Roelcke and Giovanni Maio, 309–317. Stuttgart: Steiner, 2004.

———. "Population Genetics in Israel in the 1950s: The Unconscious Internalization of Ideology." *Isis* 94, no. 4 (2003): 631–655.

Klor, Sebastian. *Between Exile and Exodus: Argentinian Jewish Immigration to Israel, 1948–1967.* Detroit: Wayne State, 2017.

Kramer, Gudrun. *A History of Palestine*. Princeton: Princeton University Press, 2008.

Kraut, Alan M. *Silent Travellers: Germs, Genes and the Immigrant Menace*. Baltimore: Johns Hopkins University Press, 1994.

Levy, Nissim. *The History of Medicine in the Holy Land: 1799–1948* [in Hebrew]. Israel: Hakibbutz Hameuhad, 1998.

Lissak, Moshe. "Images of Immigrants: Stereotypes and Stigmatization in the Period of Mass Immigration to Israel in the 1950s" [in Hebrew]. *Cathedra*, 43 (1987): 125.

———. *The Mass Immigration in the Fifties: The Failure of the Melting Pot Policy* [in Hebrew]. Jerusalem: Bialik Institute, 1999.

Little, Lester. *Plague and the End of Antiquity: The Pandemic of 541–750*. Cambridge: Cambridge University Press, 2008.

Maglen, Krista. "'The First Line of Defence': British Quarantine and the Port Sanitary Authorities in the Nineteenth Century." *Social History of Medicine* 15, no. 3 (2002): 414–428.

———. "Quarantined: Exploring Personal Accounts of Incarceration in Australian and Pacific Quarantine Stations in the Nineteenth Century." *Journal of the Royal Australian Historical Society* 91, no. 1 (2005): 1–12.

Malka, Haim. *The Selection: Selection and Discrimination in the Aliya and Absorption of Moroccan and North African Jewry 1948–1956* [in Hebrew]. Tel Aviv: Tal, 1998.

Markel, H., and A. M. Stern. "The Foreignness of Germs: The Persistent Association of Immigrants and Disease in American Society." *Milbank Quarterly* 80, no. 4 (2002): 757–788.

Markel, Howard. *Quarantine! East European Jewish Immigrants and the New York City Epidemics of 1892*. Baltimore: Johns Hopkins University Press, 1997.

Martin, Guy. "Continuity and Change in Franco-African Relations." *Journal of Modern African Studies* 33, no. 1 (1995): 1–20.

Meir-Glitzenstein, Esther. *Ben Bagdad le-Ramat Gan: Yots'ey Iraq be-Yisrael*. Jerusalem: Yad Ben-Tzvi, 2008.

Modan, Baruch, Hannah Mart, Dikla Baidatz, Ruth Steinitz, and Sheldon G. Levin. "Radiation-Induced Head and Neck Tumors." *Lancet* 303 (February 23, 1974): 277–279.

Morris, Benny. *The Birth of the Palestinian Refugee Problem Revisited*. Cambridge: Cambridge University Press, 2004.

———. "The New Historiography: Israel Confronts Its Past." *Tikkun* 3, no. 6 (1988): 19–23, 98–103.

————. *1948 and After: Israel and the Palestinians*. New York: Oxford University Press, 1994.

————. *Righteous Victims: A History of the Zionist-Arab Conflict 1881–2001*. New York: Vintage Books, 2001.

Mosse, George L. "Max Nordau, Liberalism and the New Jew." *Journal of Contemporary History* 27, no. 4 (October 1992): 565–582.

Musto, David F. "Quarantine and the Problem of AIDS." *Milbank Quarterly* 64, supp. 1 (1986): 97–117.

Naor, Mordechai. *The Atlit Camp: A Story of a Time and Place*. Israel: Atlit Heritage Site, 2010.

————. "Newspapers in the 1950's." In *The First Decade* [in Hebrew], edited by Zvi Zameret and Hana Yablonka, 215–227. Jerusalem: Yad Yitzhak Ben-Tzvi, 1997.

————. *Sefer Haaliyot: Mea Shana ve Od shel Aliya ve klita* [The book of Aliyot: One hundred years and more of Aliya and absorption]. Tel Aviv: Ministry of Defense, 1991.

Nora, Pierre. *Rethinking France. Les Lieux de Mémoire*. Vol. 1, *The State*. Chicago: University of Chicago Press, 2001.

Nordau, Max. "Muscle Jewry." In *Max Nordau to His People* [in Hebrew], edited by Benzion Netanyahu (Tel Aviv: Hotzaa Medinit, 1937).

Ofer, Dalia, ed. *Israel in the Great Wave of Immigration, 1948–1953* [in Hebrew]. Jerusalem: Yad Yitzhak Ben Tzvi, 1996.

Ohana, David. *The Origins of Israeli Mythology*. Cambridge: Cambridge University Press, 2012.

Picard, Avi. "Immigration, Health and Social Control: Medical Aspects of the Policy Governing *Aliyah* from Morocco and Tunisia, 1951–54." *Journal of Israeli History* 22, no. 2 (Autumn 2003): 33–34.

————. *Olim Be Mesora: Mediniyut Yisrael Klapey Aliyatam shel Yehudey Tzfon Africa, 1951–1956* [Cut to measure: Israel's policies regarding the *aliyah* of North African Jews, 1951–1956]. Sde Boker, Israel: Ben-Gurion University Press, 2013.

Porter, Basil, and William E. Seidelman. *The Politics of Reform in Medical Education and Health Services: The Negev Project*. New York: Springer, 1992.

Porter, Dorothy. *Health, Civilization and the State: A History of Public Health from Ancient to Modern Times*. London: Routledge, 1999.

Porter, Roy. *The Greatest Benefit to Mankind: A Medical History of Humanity*. New York: W. W. Norton, 1997.

Quarantine and Isolation: Lessons Learned from SARS. A Report to the Centers for Disease Control and Prevention. Louisville, Ky.: University of Louisville School of Medicine, 2003.

Rabinovich, Itamar, and Jehuda Reinharz, eds. *Israel in the Middle East: Documents and Readings on Society, Politics and Foreign Relations, Pre-1948 to the Present.* 2nd ed. Waltham, Mass.: Brandeis University Press, 2008.

Regev, Motti, and Edwin Seroussi. *Popular Music and National Culture in Israel.* Berkeley: University of California Press, 2004.

Reiss, Nira. *The Health Care of the Arabs in Israel (Westview Special Studies on the Middle East).* Boulder, Colo.: Westview, 1991.

Richards, Paul. *Ebola: How a People's Science Helped End an Epidemic.* London: Zed Books, 2016.

Robinson, Shira. *Citizen Strangers: Palestinians and the Birth of Israel's Liberal Settler State.* Stanford: Stanford University Press, 2013.

Roby, Bryan K. *The Mizrahi Era of Rebellion: Israel's Forgotten Civil Rights Struggle, 1948–1966.* Syracuse, N.Y.: Syracuse University Press, 2015.

Rosen, George. *A History of Public Health.* New York: MD, 1958.

Rosenberg, Charles. "Disease in History: Frames and Framers." *Milbank Quarterly* 67, no. 1 (1989): 1–15.

Rosner, Fred. "Involuntary Confinement for Tuberculosis Control: The Jewish View." *Mount Sinai Journal of Medicine* 63, no. 1 (January 1996): 44–48.

Rotenberg, Zehavit. "The Atlit Detention Camp." In *The Atlit Camp: A Story of a Time and Place*, by Mordechai Naor. Israel: Atlit Heritage Site, 2010.

Rozin, Orit. *A Home for All Jews: Citizenship, Rights, and National Identity in the New Israeli State.* Waltham, Mass.: Brandeis University Press, 2016.

———. *The Rise of the Individual in 1950s Israel: A Challenge to Collectivism.* Waltham, Mass.: Brandeis University Press, 2011.

———. "'Terms of Disgust': Hygiene and Parenthood of Immigrants from Moslem Countries as Viewed by Veteran Israelis in the 1950s" [in Hebrew]. *Iyunim Bitkumat Israel* 12 (2002): 195–238.

Rubenstein, Amnon. "The Israeli Left. 1970." In *Israel in the Middle East: Documents and Readings on Society, Politics and Foreign Relations, Pre-1948 to the Present*, edited by Itamar Rabinovich and Jehuda Reinharz. 2nd ed. Waltham, Mass.: Brandeis University Press, 2008.

Rubin, Barry. *Israel: An Introduction.* New Haven, Conn.: Yale University Press, 2012.

Rubinstein, Shimon. *The Full Collection of Articles Published by Aryeh Gelblum in "Haaretz" (13.4–6.5 1949) and the Responses to Aliya* [in Hebrew]. Illustrated by Gerti Rubinstein. Jerusalem, 2001.

Sachar, Howard. *A History of Israel from the Rise of Zionism to Our Time.* 3rd ed. New York: Knopf, 2007.

Schwartz, Barry. *Abraham Lincoln and the Forge of National Memory.* Chicago: University of Chicago Press, 2000.

———. *Abraham Lincoln in the Post-Heroic Era*. Chicago: University of Chicago Press, 2008.

Seeman, Don. *One People, One Blood: Ethiopian-Israelis and the Return to Judaism*. New Brunswick, N.J.: Rutgers University Press, 2010.

Segev, Tom. *1949: The First Israelis*. London: Free Press, 1986.

———. *The Seventh Million: The Israelis and the Holocaust*. New York: Hill and Wang, 1994.

Seidelman, Rhona. "Encounters in an Israeli Line: Shaar Ha'aliya, March 1950." *AJS Perspectives*, Fall 2014. http://perspectives.ajsnet.org/the-peoples-issue/encounters-in-an-israeli-line-shaar-ha-aliyah-march-1950/.

Seidelman, Rhona, S. Ilan Troen, and Shifra Shvarts. "'Healing' the Bodies and Souls of Immigrant Children: The Ringworm and Trachoma Institute, Shaar Ha'aliya, Israel 1952–1960." *Journal of Israeli History* 29, no. 2 (2010): 191–211.

Seidelman, William E. "Mengele Medicus: Medicine's Nazi Heritage." *Milbank Quarterly* 66, no. 2 (1988): 221–239.

———. "Nuremberg Lamentation: For the Forgotten Victims of Medical Science." *British Medical Journal* 313 (1996): 1463–1467.

Sela, Refael. "Shaar Le Aliyah oh Mahaneh Hesger?" [A gate for *Aliya* or a quarantine?]. *Haolam Hazeh*, May 31, 1951.

Shalev, Meir. *The Blue Mountain*. New York: Harper Perennial, 1991.

Shapira, Anita. "Anti-Semitism and Zionism." *Modern Judaism* 15, no. 3 (October 1995): 215–232.

———. *Israel: A History*. Waltham, Mass.: Brandeis University Press, 2014.

———, ed. *We Hereby Declare: 60 Chosen Speeches in the History of Israel* [in Hebrew]. Or Yehuda, Israel: Kinneret, Zmora-Bitan, Dvir, 2008.

Shaw, Irwin, and Robert Capa. *Report on Israel*. New York: Simon & Schuster, 1950.

Shehory-Rubin, Zipora, and Shifra Shvarts. "'*Hadassah*' *le-vri'ut ha-am: Pe'ilutah ha-bri'utit ha-hinukhit shel 'Hadassah' be-Eretz Yisrael bi-tkufat ha-mandat ha-briti*" ["Hadassah" for the health of the people: The health-education work of "Hadassah" in Eretz Israel during the British Mandate]. Jerusalem: Ha-Sifriyah ha-Tziyonit, 2003.

Shenhav, Yehuda. *The Arab Jews: A Postcolonial Reading of Nationalism, Religion, and Ethnicity*. Stanford: Stanford University Press, 2006.

Shepherd, Todd. *The Invention of Decolonization: The Algerian War and the Remaking of France*. Ithaca, N.Y.: Cornell University Press, 2006.

Shohat, Ella. "Sephardim in Israel: Zionism from the Standpoint of Its Jewish Victims." *Social Text*, no. 19/20 (Autumn 1988): 1–35.

Shvarts, Shifra. "The Birth of Israel Health Care System—an American Mother and a Russian Father." Lecture, University of North Carolina, Chapel Hill, September 2000.

———. "The Development of Mother and Infant Welfare Centers in Israel, 1854–1954." *Journal of the History of Medicine and Allied Sciences* 55, no. 4 (2000): 398–425.

———. *Health and Zionism: The Israeli Health Care System, 1948–1960.* Rochester, N.Y.: University of Rochester Press, 2008.

———. "Hospital Wars" [in Hebrew]. *Et Mol* 160, no. 2 (2001/2): 4–7.

———. "International Health and Welfare Organizations in Israel: The Early Years." In *Katyn and Switzerland: Forensic Investigators and Investigations in Humanitarian Crises, 1920–2007* [in French and English], edited by Delphine Debons, Antoine Fleury, and Jean-François Pitteloud, 325–334. Geneva: Georg, 2009.

———. *Kupat-Holim, the Histadrut and the Government* [in Hebrew]. Sde Boker, Israel: Ben-Gurion Research Center, 2000.

———. *The Workers' Health Fund in Eretz Israel: Kupat Holim, 1911–1937.* Rochester, N.Y.: University of Rochester Press, 2002.

Shvarts, Shifra, and Theodore M. Brown. "Kupat Holim, Dr. Isaac Max Rubinow and the American Zionist Medical Unit's Experiment to Establish Health Care Services in Palestine 1918–1923." *Bulletin of the History of Medicine* 72, no. 1 (1998): 28–46.

Shvarts, Shifra, Nadav Davidovitch, Rhona Seidelman, and Avishay Goldberg. "Medical Selection and the Debate over Mass Immigration in the New State of Israel (1948–1951)." *Canadian Bulletin for the History of Medicine* 22, no. 1 (2005): 5–34.

Shvarts, Shifra, and Zipora Shehory-Rubin. *Hadassah for the Health of the People—the Health Education Mission of Hadassah: The American Zionist Women in the Holy Land* [in Hebrew]. Tel Aviv: Dekel Academic, 2012.

Sikron, Moshe. "The Mass Immigration—Its Size, Characteristics and Influences." In *Immigrants and Transit Camps, 1948–1952*, edited by Mordechai Naor. Jerusalem: Yad Yitzhak Ben Zvi, 1986.

Skloot, Rebecca. *The Immortal Life of Henrietta Lacks.* New York: Broadway Books, 2011.

Smith, Andrew W. M. "Of Colonial Futures and an Administrative Alamo: Investment, Reform and the *Loi Cadre* (1956) in French West Africa." *French History* 28, no. 1 (2014): 92–113.

Somekh, Sasson. *Call It Dreaming: Memoirs 1951–2000* [in Hebrew]. Israel: Hakibbutz Hamehuad, Sifrei Siman Kriya, 2008.

Stedman, Thomas Lathrop, ed. *A Reference Handbook of the Medical Sciences*. New York: William Wood, 1917.

Sternberg, Avraham. *A People Is Absorbed*. Tel Aviv: Hakibbutz Hameuhad, 1973.

Stoler-Liss, Sachlav. "Hadrakhah ve-kidum bri'ut be-hevrot rav tarbutiyot: Ha-mikreh shel ha-aliyah ha-gedolah le-Yisrael, 1949–1956" [Health promotion and health education in multicultural societies: The case of Israeli mass immigration, 1949–1956]. PhD diss., Ben-Gurion University of the Negev, 2006.

———. "'Mothers Birth the Nation': The Social Construction of Zionist Motherhood in Wartime in Israeli Parents' Manuals." *Nashim: A Journal of Jewish Women's Studies and Gender Issues* 6 (Fall 2003): 104–118.

Stoler-Liss, Sachlav, Shifra Shvarts, and Mordechai Shani. *Lehiyot Am Hofshi Be Arzenu: Briyut Hazibur ba Aliya Ha Gdola [To Be a Healthy People in Our Land: Public Health and the Mass Immigration (1948–1960)]*. Beer Sheva, Israel: Ben-Gurion University Press.

Strange, Carolyn, and Alison Bashford, eds. *Isolation: Places and Practices of Exclusion*. London: Routledge, 2003.

Sufian, Sandra. "Arab Health Care during the British Mandate, 1920–1947." In *Separate and Cooperate, Cooperate and Separate: The Disengagement of the Palestine Health Care System from Israel and Its Emergence as an Independent System*, edited by Tamara Barnea and Rafiq Husseini, 9–31. Westport: Praeger, 2002.

———. *Healing the Land and the Nation: Malaria and the Zionist Project in Palestine, 1920–1947*. Chicago: University of Chicago Press, 2007.

Thompson, David. *Europe since Napoleon*. London: Penguin Books, 1990.

Tognotti, Eugenia. "Lessons from the History of Quarantine, from Plague to Influenza A." *Emerging Infectious Diseases* 19, no. 2 (February 2013): 254–259.

Tomes, Nancy. *The Gospel of Germs: Men, Women and the Microbe in American Life*. Cambridge, Mass.: Harvard University Press, 1999.

Troen, S. Ilan. *Imagining Zion: Dreams, Designs, and Realities in a Century of Jewish Settlement*. New Haven, Conn.: Yale University Press, 2003.

Troen, S. Ilan, and Noah Lucas, eds. *Israel: The First Decade of Independence*. Albany: State University of New York Press, 1995.

Tzahor, Zeev. "Ben-Gurion's Attitude toward the *Gola* (Diaspora) and Aliyah" [in Hebrew]. In *Kibbutz galuyot: Ha-aliyah le-Eretz Yisrael, mitos u-metzi'ut* [Ingathering of exiles: Aliyah to the land of Israel, myth, and reality], edited by Dvora Hacochen, 131–145. Jerusalem: Zalman Shazar Center for Jewish History, 1998.

Wallach, Jehuda, and Moshe Lissak, eds. *Carta's Atlas of Israel: The First Years, 1948–1961* [in Hebrew]. Jerusalem: Carta and the Israeli Ministry of Defense, 1978.

Wasserstein, Bernard. *Divided Jerusalem: The Struggle for the Holy City*. 3rd ed. New Haven, Conn.: Yale University Press, 2008.

Weindling, Paul. "The Origins of Informed Consent: The International Scientific Commission on Medical War Crimes, and the Nuremberg Code." *Bulletin of the History of Medicine* 75, no. 1 (2001): 37–71.

Weisberger, Yehuda. *Shaar Ha'aliya: The Diary of the Mass Aliya, 1947–1957* [in Hebrew]. Jerusalem: Bialik Institute, 1985.

Weiss, Meira. *The Chosen Body*. Stanford: Stanford University Press, 2002.

Weitz, Yechiam. "The Holocaust on Trial: The Impact of the Kasztner and Eichmann Trials on Israeli Society." *Israel Studies* 1, no. 2 (1996): 1–26.

———. "'Mapai' and the 'Kastner Trial.'" *Israel: The First Decade of Independence*, edited by S. Ilan Troen and Noah Lucas, 195–210. Albany: State University of New York Press, 1995.

Whelan, Richard. *Robert Capa: A Biography*. New York: Alfred A. Knopf, 1985.

Winter, Jay. *Remembering War: The Great War between Memory and History in the Twentieth Century*. New Haven, Conn.: Yale University Press, 2006.

Yablonka, Hanna. "The Development of Holocaust Consciousness in Israel: The Nuremberg, Kapos, Kastner, and Eichmann Trials." *Israel Studies* 8, no. 3 (Fall 2003): 1–24.

———. *Survivors of the Holocaust*. London: Macmillan, 1999.

Yaffe, Hillel. *Dor Maapilim: Memoirs, Journals, Letters* [in Hebrew]. Tel Aviv: Sifriyat Tarmil, 1983.

Yerushalmi, Yosef Hayim. *Zakhor: Jewish History and Jewish Memory*. New York: Schocken Books, 1982.

Zahra, Tara. *The Great Departure: Mass Migration from Eastern Europe and the Making of the Free World*. New York: Norton, 2016.

Zalashik, Rakefet. *History of Psychiatry in Palestine and Israel, 1882–1960* [in Hebrew]. Tel Aviv: Hakibbutz Hameuhad, 2008.

Zameret, Zvi. *Across a Narrow Bridge: Shaping the Education System during the Great Aliya* [in Hebrew]. Sde Boker, Israel: Ben-Gurion University of the Negev Press, 1997.

———. "Ben-Gurion and Lavon: Two Standpoints on Absorption during the Great Wave of Immigration." In *Israel in the Great Wave of Immigration, 1948–1953* [in Hebrew], edited by Dalia Ofer. Jerusalem: Yad Yitzhak Ben Tzvi, 1996.

Zameret, Zvi, and Hana Yablonka, eds. *The First Decade* [in Hebrew]. Jerusalem: Yad Yitzhak Ben-Tzvi, 1997.

Zerubavel, Yael. *Recovered Roots: Collective Memory and the Making of Israeli National Tradition*. Chicago: University of Chicago Press, 1995.

Index

Page numbers in *italics* refer to figures.

About the Author

RHONA SEIDELMAN is an assistant professor of history and the Schuster-man Chair of Israel Studies at the University of Oklahoma. She has degrees from the Hebrew University of Jerusalem and Ben-Gurion University of the Negev and has taught at Ben-Gurion University and the University of Illinois at Urbana-Champaign. Professor Seidelman is originally from Canada.